Population Policy and Reproduction in Singapore

This book examines the relationship between population policies and individual reproductive decisions in low-fertility contexts. Using the case study of Singapore, it demonstrates that the effectiveness of population policy is a function of competing notions of citizenship, and the gap between seemingly neutral policy incentives and the perceived and experienced disparate effects.

Drawing on a substantial number of personal interviews and focus groups, the book analyzes the developmental welfare state's overarching emphasis of citizen responsibility, and examines population policies that reinforce social inequalities and ignore cultural diversity. These factors combine to undermine elaborate state policy efforts in encouraging citizens' biological reproduction. The book goes on to argue that in order to facilitate positive fertility decisions, the state needs to modify the "economic production at all cost" approach and pay much more attention to the importance of social rights. This suggests that the Singapore government might profitably approach the phenomenon of very low fertility with major initiatives similar to those of other advanced industrialized societies. This book offers a significant contribution to the literature on social policy, East Asian and Southeast Asian studies.

Shirley Hsiao-Li Sun is an Assistant Professor of Sociology at Nanyang Technological University, Singapore. Her main research interests are population studies, social inequalities, citizenship and immigration, economic development and social reproduction, and science and technology.

Routledge Contemporary Southeast Asia Series

1 **Land Tenure, Conservation and Development in Southeast Asia**
Peter Eaton

2 **The Politics of Indonesia-Malaysia Relations**
One kin, two nations
Joseph Chinyong Liow

3 **Governance and Civil Society in Myanmar**
Education, health and environment
Helen James

4 **Regionalism in Post-Suharto Indonesia**
Edited by Maribeth Erb, Priyambudi Sulistiyanto and Carole Faucher

5 **Living with Transition in Laos**
Market integration in Southeast Asia
Jonathan Rigg

6 **Christianity, Islam and Nationalism in Indonesia**
Charles E. Farhadian

7 **Violent Conflicts in Indonesia**
Analysis, representation, resolution
Edited by Charles A. Coppel

8 **Revolution, Reform and Regionalism in Southeast Asia**
Cambodia, Laos and Vietnam
Ronald Bruce St John

9 **The Politics of Tyranny in Singapore and Burma**
Aristotle and the rhetoric of benevolent despotism
Stephen McCarthy

10 **Ageing in Singapore**
Service needs and the state
Peggy Teo, Kalyani Mehta, Leng Leng Thang and Angelique Chan

11 **Security and Sustainable Development in Myanmar**
Helen James

12 **Expressions of Cambodia**
The politics of tradition, identity and change
Edited by Leakthina Chau-Pech Ollier and Tim Winter

13 **Financial Fragility and Instability in Indonesia**
Yasuyuki Matsumoto

14 **The Revival of Tradition in Indonesian Politics**
The deployment of *adat* from colonialism to indigenism
Edited by Jamie S. Davidson and David Henley

15 **Communal Violence and Democratization in Indonesia**
Small town wars
Gerry van Klinken

16 **Singapore in the Global System**
Relationship, structure and change
Peter Preston

17 **Chinese Big Business in Indonesia**
The state of the capital
Christian Chua

18 **Ethno-religious Violence in Indonesia**
From soil to God
Chris Wilson

19 **Ethnic Politics in Burma**
States of conflict
Ashley South

20 **Democratization in Post-Suharto Indonesia**
Edited by Marco Bünte and Andreas Ufen

21 **Party Politics and Democratization in Indonesia**
Golkar in the post-Suharto era
Dirk Tomsa

22 **Community, Environment and Local Governance in Indonesia**
Locating the Commonwealth
Edited by Carol Warren and John F. McCarthy

23 **Rebellion and Reform in Indonesia**
Jakarta's security and autonomy polices in Aceh
Michelle Ann Miller

24 **Hadrami Arabs in Present-day Indonesia**
An Indonesia-oriented group with an Arab signature
Frode F. Jacobsen

25 **Vietnam's Political Process**
How education shapes political decision making
Casey Lucius

26 **Muslims in Singapore**
Piety, politics and policies
Kamaludeen Mohamed Nasir, Alexius A. Pereira and Bryan S. Turner

27 **Timor Leste**
Politics, history and culture
Andrea Katalin Molnar

28 **Gender and Transitional Justice**
The women of East Timor
Susan Harris Rimmer

29 **Environmental Cooperation in Southeast Asia**
ASEAN's regime for trans-boundary haze pollution
Paruedee Nguitragool

30 **The Theatre and the State in Singapore**
Terence Chong

31 **Ending Forced Labour in Myanmar**
Engaging a pariah regime
Richard Horsey

32 **Security, Development and Nation-Building in Timor-Leste**
A cross-sectoral assessment
Edited by Vandra Harris and Andrew Goldsmith

33 **The Politics of Religion in Indonesia**
Syncretism, orthodoxy, and religious contention in Java and Bali
Edited by Michel Picard and Remy Madinier

34 **Singapore's Ageing Population**
Managing healthcare and end of life decisions
Edited by Wing-Cheong Chan

35 **Changing Marriage Patterns in Southeast Asia**
Economic and socio-cultural dimensions
Edited by Gavin W. Jones, Terence H. Hull and Maznah Mohamad

36 **The Political Resurgence of the Military in Southeast Asia**
Conflict and leadership
Edited by Marcus Mietzner

37 **Neoliberal Morality in Singapore**
How family policies make state and society
Youyenn Teo

38 **Local Politics in Indonesia**
Pathways to power
Nankyung Choi

39 **Separatist Conflict in Indonesia**
The long-distance politics of the Acehnese diaspora
Antje Missbach

40 **Corruption and Law in Indonesia**
The unravelling of Indonesia's anti-corruption framework through law and legal process
Simon Butt

41 **Men and Masculinities in Southeast Asia**
Edited by Michele Ford and Lenore Lyons

42 **Justice and Governance in East Timor**
Indigenous approaches and the 'new subsistence state'
Rod Nixon

43 **Population Policy and Reproduction in Singapore**
Making future citizens
Shirley Hsiao-Li Sun

Population Policy and Reproduction in Singapore

Making future citizens

Shirley Hsiao-Li Sun

Routledge
Taylor & Francis Group
LONDON AND NEW YORK

First published 2012
by Routledge
2 Park Square, Milton Park, Abingdon, Oxon OX14 4RN

Simultaneously published in the USA and Canada
by Routledge
711 Third Avenue, New York, NY 10017

Routledge is an imprint of the Taylor & Francis Group, an informa business

British Library Cataloguing in Publication Data
A catalogue record for this book is available from the British Library

Library of Congress Cataloging-in-Publication Data
Sun, Shirley Hsiao-Li.
Population policy and reproduction in Singapore : making future citizens / Shirley Hsiao-Li Sun.
p. cm. — (Routledge contemporary Southeast Asia series ; 43)
Includes bibliographical references and index.
1. Singapore—Population policy. 2. Family policy—Singapore. 3. Fertility, Human—Singapore. I. Title. II. Series: Routledge contemporary Southeast Asia series ; 43.
HB3645.A3S86 2011
363.9095957—dc23 2011025864

ISBN: 978–0–415–67068–5 (hbk)
ISBN: 978–0–203–14618–7 (ebk)

Typeset in Times New Roman
by Swales & Willis Ltd, Exeter, Devon

MIX
Paper from responsible sources
FSC® C004839

Printed and bound in Great Britain by the MPG Books Group

For my loved ones

Contents

Figures

Tables

Acknowledgments

I owe many people my deepest appreciation. The following paragraphs gratefully acknowledge just some of those colleagues and friends. I have a special indebtedness to Troy Duster, whose astute observations and penetrating theories of complex human behavior have invaluably raised the level of the investigation at critical junctures. His wisdom, foresight, humor, and unfailing support have been vital in the completion of this project.

For reviews of all or portions of this manuscript, I thank the anonymous reviewers and my colleagues, Hong Liu, Kian Woon Kwok and Francis Khek Gee Lim in particular, at Nanyang Technological University in Singapore. Additionally, I would like to thank Kyung-Sup Chang, Beng-Huat Chua, Mary Daly, Gavin Jones, Susan A. McDaniel, Emiko Ochiai, Ito Peng, Mika Toyota, Biao Xiang, Mui-Ting Yap, Wei-Jun Jean Yeung, and Yanxia Zhang, for their insightful, challenging and always-helpful feedback and encouragement.

Portions of this book were presented at numerous conferences and seminars and I am grateful for the questions and comments I received at each. Drafts of Chapter 1 were presented at the Care Regimes in Asia conference organized by the Kyoto University Global Center of Excellence Program (Japan) and the Sociology of Reproduction panel for the Eastern Sociological Society (USA). An early draft of Chapter 4 was presented at the Asian Social Protection in Comparative Perspective international conference co-organized by the Association for Public Policy Analysis and Management, University of Maryland School of Public Policy (USA) and the Lee Kuan Yew School of Public Policy at the National University of Singapore. Sections of this book were also presented at seminars and conferences organized by the Asia Research Institute and at the annual meetings of the American Sociological Association, the Canadian Sociological Association, the International Sociological Association and the Association for Asian Studies on the Pacific Coast. For permission to quote from published materials, I would like to thank Baywood Publishing Co., Inc., and Joel P. Rubin, the editor of the *Journal of Workplace Rights*.

I am indebted to the utmost professional, clear and careful guidance of the editors at Routledge, Dorothea Schaefter, Leanne Hinves, and Jillian Morrison.

My appreciation also goes to the Singapore Ministry of Education and the Nanyang Technological University for the research grant. Excellent research assistance was provided by Hemavalli Singaram Padmanathan, Ha Pham Doan Trang, Filzah Armalia Rahmat, Emily Cheah, Eunice Chia, Delia Phua, Shivali Nayak, Jing Ying Tay, Joanna Lee, Hui Hoon Chan, Ying Lan Wong, Siti Ramziyain Ramdzan, and Dylan Ming Hui Loh.

Of course, this project would not have been possible without the generosity and kindness of all 221 Singaporeans who shared their rich experiences, views, and opinions. It is my hope that their voices will be heard. My heartfelt thanks also go to Annie Park, Tony Park, Eleanor Yeh, Tom Lai, and Junmin Wang, who have provided all-round good cheer. Finally, I want to thank my parents, Chen-Feng Shen and Bin Sun, for their love and support, and my son, Alexander, whose high expectation fueled more hours of work when sheer force of will did not.

1 Introduction

Making future citizens

Citizenship, in theory and practice, provides a means of exploring the relationship between the state and the individual. It also provides a framework for considering the aims and outcomes of public policy. Recently, scholars have called for more empirical work in the field of citizenship studies (Conover *et al.* 1991; Lister 1997, 2003; Desforges *et al.* 2005; Isin *et al.* 2008). This book is an attempt to make a contribution to the field through an empirical investigation of the relationship between state population policies and individual childbearing decisions. The need to take seriously individuals' perceptions and experiences of state policies gains greater urgency in the context of a potential conflict of interest between the state and citizens regarding human reproduction—a matter of fundamental significance in governance and personal life. As will be shown, social inequalities (e.g., class, gender, and race) are not merely objective realities that the state passively manages and regulates. States also actively constitute the very object that they seek to manage and regulate, and part of the analytical task is to specify mechanisms adopted in a given nation-state. This constitutive act then necessarily generates questions about the issues of citizens' rights and responsibilities, and the role of the state in social provision. In the larger context of the nation-state's response to global capitalism, what is the relationship between a particular conceptualization of citizenship and the employment status of citizens? Should citizenship status confer rights independent of an individual's socio-economic standing? In the public sphere, who is the idealized citizen?

T. H. Marshall (1950) advanced the "citizenship-as-rights" thesis within the context of the historical rise of industrial capitalism. Britain was a dominant imperial and colonial power during the eighteenth to twentieth centuries, and the nation-state was the key institutional actor (Chandler 1990). In sharp contrast, the last few decades have witnessed an ever-expanding global capitalism,[1] with increasing cross-border labor migration[2] and volatile transnational movement of capital.[3] In this book, I explore the relationship between state and citizenry under these shifting conditions. In some countries, the government attempts to steer a viable course in the face of global capitalism, rather than in the context of industrial capitalism. Here, the state is more aptly characterized as a "developmental welfare state" (Goodman *et al.* 1998; Midgley and Tang 2001; Ramesh 2004), and a "productivist welfare state" (Gough *et al.* 2004; Holliday 2000, 2005; Holliday and Wilding

2004), with social policies designed to help the nation better integrate into, and excel in, the global capitalist order. The conceptualization of citizenship, in this instance, tends to emphasize citizen duties and responsibilities.

I suggest that the developmental and productivist thesis finds its fullest expression in the transformation of Singapore, a city-state of 5.08 million in 2010, with a per capita Gross Domestic Product (GDP) of US$43,117, exceeding that of Japan (US$42,820) (International Monetary Fund 2011).[4] As will be further elaborated in Chapter 3, the city-state not only emphasizes citizenship-as-responsibility but, in tandem, adopts the citizens-as-human resources paradigm, which has been seen by scholars and policy makers as the key to its economic success and growing international prominence (see, for example, Low and Johnston 2003; Osman-Gani 2004; Sung 2006; Wan and Hui 2008). However, there are limits to the logic of the "citizenship-as-responsibility" and "human-resources economic-development" paradigms. While scholars of citizenship studies do not theorize on population policies and their effects, this book presents substantial empirical evidence indicating that the gap between the aim of three decades of pronatalist population policies (i.e., government policies that are designed to encourage childbearing) and the outcome of persistent low fertility in the globalized city-state of Singapore, is a function of competing notions of citizenship and the role of the state in social provisions.

According to the United Nations (2010):

> today, 42 per cent of the world's population lives in low-fertility countries, that is, countries where women are not having enough children to ensure that, on average, each woman is replaced by a daughter who survives to the age of procreation.

Indeed, along with their counterparts in Europe, several post-industrial societies in Asia have entered an era of below-replacement fertility (i.e., less than 2.1 children per woman of childbearing age). For instance, the total fertility rates (TFR) for Japan, South Korea, Hong Kong, Taiwan, and Singapore for 2010 were estimated at 1.3, 1.2, 1.0, 1.0, and 1.2 respectively (Population Reference Bureau 2010). Governments in these countries have attempted to address the issue of declining fertility by adopting a variety of population policy measures to encourage the local population to give birth to more children. However, as Jones *et al.* (2009a) noted, "existing pro-natalist policies do not appear to be having much effect in these countries, and although governments realize that more needs to be done to encourage fertility, exactly *what* should be done remains elusive" (emphasis in original).

Singapore is a significant research site for the investigation of the relationship between state population policies and individual childbearing decisions for three primary reasons. First, Singapore is the developmental and productivist state par excellence (Lee 2007). Second, as Table 1.1 shows, Singapore was the first country in the Pacific Asia region to reverse earlier anti-natalist policies (Jones *et al.* 2009b). Third, pronatalist concerns have constantly remained a top priority in Singapore's public policy making, which has arrived at a multi-pronged approach that the government revisits and fine-tunes on a regular basis. The campaign "Have Three, Or More [Children] If You Can Afford It" was launched in 1987, and the "Baby Bonus" Scheme was introduced in 2000. Recent expansions of pronatalist policy initiatives first took effect in 2004, and then in August 2008. However, in spite of such governmental policy efforts, Singapore's TFR reached a historic low of 1.16 babies per resident female in 2010, compared with 1.83 in 1990, and 1.6 in 2000. How can we better understand the gap between the stated policy goal—"bringing Singapore's population growth back to the replacement level of 2.1 children per woman" (Ministry of Education, Singapore 2007)—and the outcome of persistent low fertility?

To answer this vital question, the book advances an alternative theoretical lens—citizenship—through which to understand state population policies and their effects. Moreover, I draw on qualitative data obtained through extensive semi-structured personal interviews and focus-group discussions with Singaporean citizens, the supposed beneficiaries of state pronatalist incentives (permanent residents are not eligible for such benefits).[5] The goal is to historicize such policies and offer a fuller context for reproductive decisions. This book is, therefore, distinct from, and complementary to, existing literature based on content analysis of population policy or statistical analysis of large-scale surveys.

In what follows, I first provide a succinct overview of the issue of rights and responsibilities (and the relationship between the two) that is central to the institution of citizenship. While the issue is not new, it has received more scholarly attention as the neo-liberal approach to governance has gained ascendance (Bezanson 2006; Brodie 1997, 2007; Faulks 1998, 2000b; Isin 2008). I also highlight the call for an understanding of citizenship as a lived experience. A specific approach to citizenship then entails particular demands on the state. Thus, I draw on the developmental welfare state and productivist welfare state literature and highlight the role of the family in providing "welfare" in East Asia.[6] Third, I describe demographic transitions

Table 1.1 Delays in reversing anti-natalist policies, selected East Asian countries

Country	*Years in which replacement fertility was reached*	*Year in which anti-natalist policy was reversed*	*Comments*
Singapore	1975	1987	
South Korea	1984	1996	Very mildly pronatalist policies
South Korea	1984	2004	More serious pronatalist measures
Taiwan	1984	1992	Pronatalist statement but no measures
Taiwan	1984	2006	Specific pronatalist measures under consideration
Japan	1973	1990	Mildly pronatalist measures
China	1992	No reversal	25 percent below replacement in 2007, policy not altered

Source: Adapted from Table 1.2 in Jones *et al.* (2009).

in developmental states—characterized as "compressed modernity" by Chang (1999)—where the period between two fertility declines (when the fertility rate was stable, and at around replacement level) was almost nonexistent.[7] Lastly, I turn to the city-state of Singapore, which leads the way toward a pronatalist policy revolution in the newly industrialized countries in Asia and among the less-developed regions. In summary, this book hopes to illustrate how social reproduction in the contemporary context of "lowest-low fertility" (Kohler, Billari, and Ortega 2002) in advanced Asian countries can be fruitfully studied as a site to reveal shifting trajectories of citizenship at different stages of nation-building.

The central theoretical framework: citizenship

To begin, the most influential exposition of the conception of citizenship-as-rights is T. H. Marshall's *Citizenship and Social Class* (1950). Marshall argues that civil, political, and social elements define the institution of citizenship:

> The civil element is composed of the rights necessary for individual freedom—liberty of the person, freedom of speech, thought and faith, the right to own property and to conclude valid contracts, and the right to justice. The last is of a different order from the others, because it is the right to defend and assert all one's rights on terms of equality with others and by due process of law. . . . By the political element I mean the right to participate in the exercise of political power, as a member of a body. . . By the social element I mean the whole range from the right to a modicum of economic welfare and security to the right to share to the full in the social heritage and to live the life of a civilized being according to the standards prevailing in the society.
>
> (Marshall 1950: 10–11)

This interpretation of citizenship-as-rights is closely associated with the welfare state. As Bussemaker and Voet (1998: 287) noted: "it was T. H. Marshall who finally laid out the map for post-World War citizenship notions in which social and liberal notions were reconciled through the community, e.g., the welfare state." The larger historical context of Marshall's approach to citizenship is industrial capitalism, and Marshall (1950: 77) suggested, "the preservation of economic inequality has been made more difficult by the enrichment of the status of citizenship." Indeed, Mau (2004: 64) noted that:

> in the ideal universal welfare regime the promotion of equality is an end in itself. The overarching goal of such forms of provision—the objective of providing decommodified welfare for all citizens—derives from the understanding of the responsibilities of the larger collectivity.

There are, however, significant variations in welfare-state regimes. For instance, in Esping-Andersen's canonical formulation (1990), there are liberal, corporatist, and social democratic welfare states.

Feminist critiques have shed light on how the welfare state itself is patriarchal (Pateman 1988), how the provision of welfare is organized through families as well as through states and markets (Orloff 1993), how "the state is not a uniform structure that acts to impose a singular set of expectations on women . . . [but] a network of differentiated institutions, layered with conflicting and competing messages about gender" (Haney 1996), and how the working mother is the privileged subject of gendered welfare regime studies (Brush 2002). They have also pointed out that the central relationship between individual and state is not solely between paid work and welfare, but also between paid work, welfare, and unpaid work (Taylor-Gooby 1991). Bussemaker and Voet (1998: 288) summarized the feminist contribution thus:

> Studies focusing on the relation between care, gender and citizenship have raised the critical questions of whether and to what extent care, especially in the private sphere, tends to exclude women from social citizenship, and whether care work should be recognized as a basis for citizenship rights, for example through care allowances.

There are, however, disagreements in the literature about whether there are different kinds of citizenship with corresponding variable notions of entitlement to the state's goods and services as rights. For example, on the one hand, Turner (2001: 189) demonstrated that there are different models of citizenship and argued that "effective entitlement was based on participation in work, war, and reproduction, resulting in three types of social identity: worker-citizens, warrior-citizens, and parent-citizens." Turner (2010: 243) further emphasized that "the citizen who enjoys the provision of goods and who has entitlements must also be engaged in various public and private spaces. Without this crucial component [participation], the entitled citizen may well be a passive subject." On the other hand, Somers (2008) is critical of how entitlements have come to be linked predominantly to paid employment in the United States, excluding the unemployed and immigrants. Drawing on the instance of poor and African-American citizens abandoned after hurricane Katrina, she demonstrated how formal citizenship failed under the rising influence of neo-liberal market fundamentalism. Somers argued, instead, that "citizenship is the right to have rights" (2008: xiv).

Furthermore, the modern reality of multiethnic and multicultural societies underscores another important debate between individual and group rights (Kymlicka and Norman 1994). Schuck (2002: 135) wrote, "profound tensions arise . . . when the state accords legal rights or duties to groups qua group that may override those of individuals, or when it grounds individuals' rights or duties on their group membership." Ironically, however, there are valid reasons why group-based rights are required in order to achieve the universality of inclusion and participation of everyone embedded in the liberal notion of citizenship. Young (1989: 251) highlighted two reasons, in particular. On the one hand, "the idea of citizenship as expressing a general will has tended to enforce homogeneity of citizens," and "in practice excluded groups judged not capable of adopting that general point of view."

On the other hand, "where differences in capacities, culture, values, and behavioral styles exist among groups, but some of these groups are privileged, strict adherence to a principle of equal treatment tends to perpetuate oppression or disadvantage." Under these circumstances, there is a need to facilitate inclusion and participation of all citizens in political life by "the articulation of special rights that attend to group differences." In other words, theoretically, group-differentiated citizenship or group-specific rights engender consequences that can be evaluated in light of arguably different political objectives. The real challenge, as alluded to above, is to examine the theoretical debate within empirical contexts.

Citizenship as a lived experience

It is important to recognize that citizenship is not just about rights and responsibilities, but also status attainment and national identity. There are at least three dimensions of citizenship: status (formal state membership and the rules of access to it); rights (formal capacities and immunities connected with such status); and, finally, identity (social integration and national belonging). In terms of the status dimension, Joppke (2008) emphasized that, in Western Europe, access to citizenship was liberalized in the second half of the twentieth century. As for social rights, which were traditionally guaranteed in national welfare states with relatively homogeneous populations, Joppke noted that minority rights have gained prominence. Liberalized access to citizenship and the increased emphasis on minority rights over social rights have implications on the identity dimension: "the space for the re-nationalization of citizenship is limited by norms of equality and non-discrimination, which allow only universalistic answers to the question of identity." More importantly, regarding the "identity" aspect of citizenship, Joppke (2008: 43) suggested that:

> Citizenship as identity has two possible meanings: the actual views held by ordinary people; and official views propagated by the state. What ordinary people associate with citizenship is one of the biggest lacunae in the literature.

A common method of investigation that reveals the direction of change in citizenship is critical policy analysis (Cox 1998; Dwyer 1998; Faulks 1998, 2000b), and there exists a rich body of literature suggesting an increasing emphasis on citizenship-duties, dating back to the 1990s (Plant 1991). Handler (2003: 230) analyzed changes in labor market policies in both Western Europe and the US, arguing that a "fundamental change" had occurred in which "social citizenship is changed from status to contract." As Handler noted, "social benefits are rights that attach by virtue of status – the status of citizenship. Under the new regime, benefits have become conditional, rights attach only if obligations are fulfilled" (ibid.).

In Canada, Brodie (1997, 2007) eloquently argued that "social citizenship is being eclipsed by market citizenship." Drawing on the Canadian experience, Brodie articulated that:

> The neo-liberal state's meso-discourse of performativity is especially challenging for women and all equity-seeking groups because it prescribes the ascendancy of market relations over political negotiation or ethical considerations. . . . By performativity I mean that state practices are increasingly being formulated within the terms of the market. *The neo-liberal state is fashioning itself as a market player rather than as the purveyor of public goods or as the instrument of the democratic will.*
>
> (Brodie 1997: 223–225, my emphasis)

Schild (2000: 282) demonstrated that, in Chile's emerging "market citizenship" and neo-liberal governance, "state agents are translators on the one hand of official documents into instances of participatory learning and empowerment, and on the other of people's realities into instances of documentary categories of poverty." Dwyer (2002: 291–292) found that, in Great Britain:

> there is a view [among focus group participants] that the state should continue to play a direct role in future welfare provision; the degree to which individuals are willing to accept the principle of conditional welfare rights depends extensively on the context of its imposition; a substantial number of citizens see the imposition of certain limits to welfare provision . . . as a legitimate part of the citizenship package.

Bezanson (2006) explored the "dual-earner female-carer model" and the experiences of household insecurity that emerged in relation to the Conservative government's neo-liberal restructuring in Canada.

It is important, however, for the issue of social citizenship to be taken up, not exclusively through analysis of "law and policy in books," but also "law and policy in action" (Conover 1991; Desforges *et al.* 2005; Siltanen 2002). Hall and Williamson (1999: 2) suggested that the notion of *lived citizenship* "refers to the meaning that citizenship actually has in people's lives and the ways in which people's social and cultural background and material circumstances affect their lives as citizens." Lister (2007) suggested the importance of studying the cultural, social, and political practices that constitute "lived citizenship for different groups of citizens in different national and spatial contexts." Isin *et al.* (2008: 11) illustrated the importance of "recasting the social in citizenship" through "an analysis of social relations at various scales and sites" to reveal how social groups are constructed and/or privileged.

This book complements recent studies, conducted, for the most part, in Western countries, that aim to understand social processes and lived experiences under a neoliberal citizenship regime, with its attendant state emphasis on citizen-responsibility. In Asian contexts, Wong and Wong (2005: 19), drawing on an attitude survey, showed that "universal ideals of social citizenship have strong appeal among the Chinese in Hong Kong, even though the latter are conventionally seen as having low expectations in the area of social rights." Wong, Wang, and Kaun (2009: 59) found that, in surveys conducted in Hong Kong and Taiwan, "social citizenship rights do not lose their momentum despite the strong traditional values of responsibility, family, and self-reliance." Indeed, as I shall argue, the phenomenon of persistent below-replacement fertility, despite state efforts, is intricately linked to the notion of social citizenship.

The developmental and productivist welfare state in Asia

The larger problematique of the book is the relationship between state and citizens, with particular attention paid to *lived citizenship*. Moreover, this study explores the interconnections of state population policies and individual fertility behavior as a site of investigation, not least because the making of future citizens is a joint enterprise—the reproduction of the nation at the state level, and family planning at the individual level. The empirical puzzle is the divergent phenomena of Singapore's three-decade-long history of pronatalist policies and its persistent decline in fertility rates. Before we proceed, however, it is necessary to understand that in East Asia, as White and Goodman (1998:14–15) have suggested, post-war Japan, South Korea, Taiwan, Hong Kong, and Singapore are "developmental welfare states," with common elements:

> At one level they reflect the broader East Asian pattern of state-sponsored development, whereby welfare arrangements have been shaped to fit the strategic priority of rapid industrialization. Rather than being "wasted" on "unproductive" welfare expenditures, financial resources have been concentrated on economic development; governments have sought to keep expenditures on social assistance down and to design funded systems of social insurance which could also provide financial resources for investment in industry and infrastructure. In consequence, these might be called "developmental welfare systems." . . . Welfare programmes were overwhelmingly introduced by those in power rather than as a result of popular demand. The motives of those in power have focused on the priority of rapid industrialization, partly for reasons of domestic stability and partly in response to geopolitical pressures, notably the need to compete with threatening neighbors in a Cold War world.

More recently, Holliday (2000, 2005) advanced the term "productivism" and "productivist welfare state" to describe the state's social provisions in East Asia, including Singapore. Holliday (2005: 148) suggested that "social policy is an extension of economic policy, and is subordinated to and defined by economic objectives." To the extent that the goal of the state's social investment is to enable citizens to become more productive economically, I find that productivism captures the essence of the relationship between economic, social, and population policies, as we shall see in the chapters that follow. In general, I suggest that "developmentalism" and "productivism" draw our attention to the discussion of means and ends of state social provisions; to put it more concisely, the state may be said to be a developmentalist and productivist welfare state when social expenditures are aimed primarily at developing citizens' human capital to strengthen their economic productivity. Table 1.2 illustrates the comparatively low government expenditures on social provisions—such as education, health, social security and welfare, and housing—as percentages of Gross Domestic Products in selected Asian countries.

Concurrently, as Esping-Andersen (2001) pointed out, in East Asia, "familialism" characterizes welfare provision—that is, the institution of the family has assumed "the bulk of welfare responsibility towards its members, in terms of both income distribution and care provision." Ochiai (2010) illustrated the inadequacy of reducing welfare regimes in Asia through simple categories such as the "Asian model" or "familialism," highlighting diversity in patterns of care provision in different Asian societies. Nevertheless, Ochiai (ibid.) argued that "unlike the second fertility decline in Europe, which was said to be driven by individualism, the lowest-

Table 1.2 Share of government expenditure on social policies

Percentage of Gross Domestic Products	*1990*	*2007*	*2008*	*2009*
South Korea				
Education	2.92	3.12	3.72	3.66
Health	n.a.	0.2	0.22	0.27
Social security & welfare	1.28	4.27	4.64	5.08
Housing & community amenities	0.15	1.47	1.35	1.6
TOTAL	n.a.	9.06	9.93	10.61
Hong Kong				
Education	2.77	3.33	4.48	3.6
Health	1.54	2.08	2.19	2.37
Social security & welfare	8.86	2.16	2.34	2.51
Housing & community amenities	3.46	2.03	3.99	2.68
TOTAL	16.63	9.6	13	11.16
Japan				
Education	3.54	3.78	3.82	n.a.
Health	4.47	7.19	7.43	n.a.
Social security & welfare	7.4	12.25	12.84	n.a.
Housing & community amenities	0.3	0.33	0.31	n.a.
TOTAL	15.71	23.55	24.4	n.a.
Singapore				
Education	4.02	2.88	3.05	n.a.
Health	0.93	0.84	1.01	n.a.
Social security & welfare	0.43	0.56	2.01	n.a.
Housing & community amenities	1.24	1.69	1.2	n.a.
TOTAL	6.62	5.97	7.27	n.a.
Taiwan (Taipei, China)				
Education	0.97	1.63	1.7	n.a.
Health	0.14	0.19	0.2	n.a.
Social security & welfare	2.76	3.24	3.25	n.a.
Housing & community amenities	0.3	0.32	0.24	n.a.
TOTAL	4.17	5.38	5.39	n.a.

Source: Asian Development Bank (2010).

low fertility in East Asia is a result of familialism." To understand the relationship between South Korea's political economic development and the institution of the family, Chang and Song (2010: 539) suggested that "South Korean families have functioned as a highly effective receptacle for the country's highly compressed conditions of modernity and late modernity." Indeed, Chang (1999) noted that no South Korean administration had shown serious commitment to the provision of social safety nets for people with severe material, physical, and psychological needs. Thus, "the plummeting fertility rate . . . [does] not attest to any fundamental transition to individualist society, but, rather . . . manifest[s] the continuing primacy of institutionalized familism in South Korea" (Chang 2010b: 26).

Two demographic transitions

Like varying models of welfare provisions conditioned by historical and structural circumstances, there are also "two demographic transitions" (Ness and Low 2000). Demographic transition is defined as the change in a population (or society) from high to low birth and death rates. As Ness and Low (ibid.: 25–29) described:

> The "past" demographic transition occurred more gradually from lower original levels, bringing slower rates of population growth . . . Though the dates and rates of change varied considerably, all of Europe and Russia, North America, Australia, New Zealand and Japan went from high birth and death rates of traditional, rural-agrarian societies, to the low birth and death rates of modern, urban-industrial societies. The last of the MDRs [more developed regions] to complete this past demographic transition was Japan, in which fertility began falling slowly in the 1920s, then dropped precipitously after the World War II.

In stark contrast, "the current demographic transition [in Asia, Africa and Latin America] is moving more rapidly than the past, involves far greater numbers, and is driven by distinctive new, bureaucratically portable, technologies, which help to control both mortality and fertility" (ibid.: 29). Ochiai (2010) and Chang (1999) emphasized that the demographic transition in Asia has its own characteristic; as Ochiai put it:

> If we think of the period between these two fertility declines—when the fertility rate was stable and at around the replacement level—as the "golden age" of First Modernity, then the length of this period was about 50 years in Europe and America, 20 years in Japan, and almost nonexistent in the rest of Asia. As the Asian societies other than Japan have not experienced a stable First Modernity, they have plunged headlong and directly into Second Modernity. (2010: 8)

Indeed, Bloom and Williamson (1998: 419) wrote definitively that "the demographic transition has been more dramatic in East Asia [including China, Hong

Kong (China), Japan, the Republic of Korea, Singapore and Taiwan (China)] during the twentieth century than in any other region or historical period." More importantly, public policy has played an important role in the current demographic transition (Caldwell and Caldwell 1996); or as Ness and Ando (1984) put it, these countries are engaged in an "anti-natalist policy revolution." The present condition of low-fertility in these countries is shown in Table 1.3. These countries could perhaps be said to lead the "pro-natalist policy revolution."

Population, state, and citizenship in Singapore

The picture of Singapore's population is, to say the least, changing rapidly. Singapore completed its demographic transition in the mid-1970s, as Figure 1.1 shows. The total fertility rate has decreased from 6.55 in 1947, to 4.62 in 1965, to 2.08 (replacement level) in 1975, and has been below replacement level since 1977. "Resident TFR for the Chinese (1.08) remained lower than that for Malays (1.82) and Indians (1.14) in 2009" (Singapore Department of Statistics 2009).

Moreover, as shown in Table 1.4, as in other post-industrial societies, in addition to declining fertility rates, Singapore is experiencing a decreasing marriage rate, but a rising median age at first marriage and rising divorce rates.

Despite declining fertility rates, as can be seen in the same table, the size of the population has grown dramatically in a few decades, from 2.07 million in 1970 to 4.99 million in 2009. The Chinese formed 74 percent of the resident population. The Malay and Indian share stood at 13 percent and 9.2 percent respectively. Immigration policy has gradually become a key component in the government's efforts to sustain population growth, which is deemed to be of central importance for the country's economic development. As the table illustrates, while total population has grown, the percentage of resident population has declined from 97 percent in 1970 to 75 percent in 2009. Among 5.08 million recorded in the June

Table 1.3 Total fertility rates of selected countries

Country	*Year*	*Rate*	*Year*	*Rate*
China	1970	5.7	2001	1.4
Denmark	1970	2.0	2001	1.7
France	1970	2.5	1999	1.8
Finland	1970	1.8	2001	1.7
Italy	1970	2.4	2000	1.2
Japan	1970	2.1	2000	1.3
Korea	1970	4.3	2000	1.5
Norway	1970	2.5	2001	1.8
Singapore	1970	3.1	2000	1.7
Sweden	1970	1.9	2001	1.6
Spain	1970	2.9	2000	1.2
United Kingdom	1972	2.2	2000	1.6
United States	1970	2.5	2000	2.1

Source: Population Division, Department of Economic and Social Affairs, United Nations (2004).

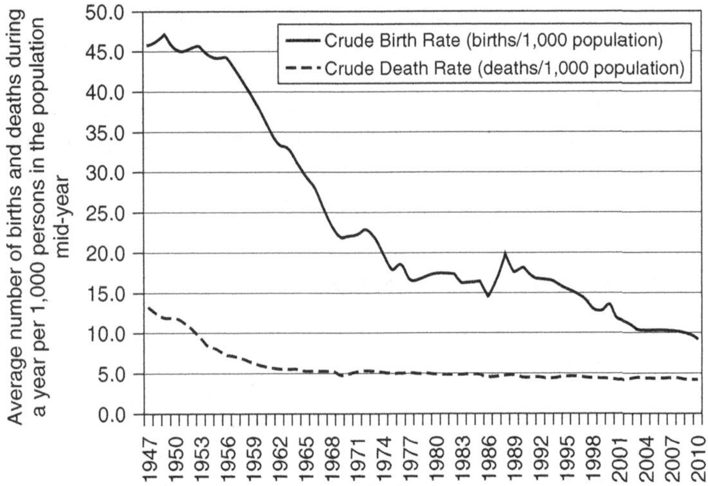

Figure 1.1 Demographic transition in Singapore

Sources: Sandhu and Wheatley (1989); Saw (1980); Singapore Department of Statistics (2009a, 2010c).

2010 census, were 3.77 million Singapore residents (3.23 million Singapore citizens and 541,000 permanent residents), and 1.31 million foreigners (including 1.05 million on various types of work visas, and 0.26 million on long-term dependent visas).

Singapore has been characterized and analyzed as a developmental state (Chua 2007; Rodan 1989; Rodan, Hewison, and Robison 2006; Sung 2006; Tremewan 1994), a productivist state (Holliday 2000), and a social investment state (Pereira 2008). What these various scholarly, analytical characterizations have in common is the suggestion that there is a set of state practices and domestic institutions integral to Singapore's economic transformation—most notably the Central Provident Fund (CPF) and Housing Development Board (HDB)—which developed, historically, as institutional responses to pressing issues of worker retirement pensions and housing shortages. Turnbull, in her historical account of how the People's Action Party [PAP] met the challenge of Singapore's "unanticipated independence" from Malaysia, wrote, "all the PAP leaders were pragmatists . . . the party took pride in rejecting not merely communism but ideologies in general, in the belief that people wanted good government in the solid shape of jobs, housing, schools, and healthcare" (2009: 272–274). Nonetheless, Hill and Lian (1995: 1) showed how citizenship in Singapore was conceived as conferring "duties" in the stage of nation-creation, notably "in a state which has firmly rejected welfarism, and whose political leaders have constantly maintained that the values of the collectivity over those of autonomous individuals are essential to its very survival."

In terms of its developmental and productivist character, first, correlating to the idea that social policies cater to economic development needs, and that "[social] investment implies return," the Singaporean government pays particular attention

Table 1.4 Key demographic indicators in Singapore

	1970	*1980*	*1990*	*2000*	*2009*
Total population ('000)	2074.5	2413.9	3047.1	4027.9	4987.6
Resident population ('000)	2013.6	2282.1	2735.9	3273.4	3733.9
Resident population (percentage)	97.06	94.54	89.79	81.27	74.86
Singapore citizen population ('000)	1874.8	2194.3	2623.7	2985.9	3200.7
Singapore citizen population (percentage in resident population)	93.1	96.15	95.9	91.22	85.72
Singapore permanent resident population ('000)	138.8	87.8	112.1	287.5	533.2
Singapore permanent resident population (percentage in resident population)	6.9	3.85	4.1	8.78	14.28
Density (total population per sq km)	3538	3907	4814	5900	7022
Total marriages[a]	14572	22444	23953	22561	26081
General marriage rate[a,b]					
Males (per 1000 unmarried resident males)	51.6	55.0	52.6	48.1	43.6
Females (per 1000 unmarried resident females)	67.3	68.9	60.9	49.9	41.1
Median age at first marriage[a,c] (years)					
Grooms	26.9	26.7	28.0	28.7	29.8
Brides	23.1	23.6	25.3	26.2	27.5
Total divorces & annulments	N.A.	1721	3634	5160	7386
General divorce rate[d]					
Males (per 1000 married resident males)	N.A.	3.7	6.1	6.5	7.7
Females (per 1000 married resident females)	N.A.	3.8	6.1	6.5	7.3
Total live births	45934	41217	51142	46997	39570
Resident live births	N.A.	40100	49787	44765	36925
Crude birth rate[e] (per 1000 population)	22.1	17.6	18.2	13.7	9.9
Total fertility rate[e] (per female)	3.07	1.82	1.83	1.60	1.22

Source: Singapore Department of Statistics (2009a, 2010a)

Notes:

a Excludes marriages previously solemnized outside Singapore or under religious and customary rites.

b Rates for 1970 and 1980 are based on total marriages and total population.

c Refer to total marriages.

d Includes annulments. Data on divorces and annulments from 2004 onwards have been revised to be based on residents. Resident population comprises Singapore Citizens and Permanent Residents.

e Data refer to Singapore residents. For 1970, data refer to total population.

to education. The state began providing mass education during the periods of industrial transformation (1965–1980) and industrial upgrading (1980–2000), which helped produce requisite human resources to support the economy. Indeed, according to Singapore's Ministry of Education (2009), there is no school fee for primary school students and fees for secondary school students are low, except in the case of "autonomous" and "independent schools," which collect their own fees.

In addition, there are government subsidies for education, most notably the Edusave Scheme, which "rewards students who perform well or who make good progress in their academic and non-academic work, and provides students and schools with funds to pay for enrichment programmes or to purchase additional resources." It is noteworthy, however, that tuition, textbooks, and other miscellaneous expenditures are not included under this state-funded scheme, and the government sets the criteria for Edusave usage. This is an example of state subsidies being tied to performance and merit, an embodiment of the "return on investment" principle.

Second, in addition to the idea of the integration of economic and social dimensions, the primary role of the developmental state is to provide opportunities. The most prominent example of this in Singapore's context might be the government's overriding concern with creating employment opportunities. Unemployment rates have generally been kept below 5 percent. Another example might be free education for Singaporean-Malays. As Lai (2002) reported:

> the Singapore Government has interpreted its constitutional duty as providing opportunities for Malays to compete on equal terms with the rest of the population by providing assistance wherever needed. This has, largely, been in the field of education, where up until recently, free education for Malays was one of the cornerstones of the Government's policy.

However, in June 1990, the government announced the end of the automatic waiver of fees for tertiary education for Malays (Minorities at Risk Project, Chronology for Malays in Singapore 2004).

Third, in terms of the focus on economic contribution, the CPF is, essentially, a comprehensive social security savings scheme in which employed citizens and their employers make monthly contributions. As Low (2004: 308) argued, the "CPF is a lynchpin in the developmental Singapore Inc. ensemble." Moreover, "generally, the paternalistic government prefers wealth transfer through housing and assets rather than income transfer. Social welfare payments are intentionally minimal with jobs available." Indeed, Low and Johnston (2003: 217) noted, "[the] self-financing Central Provident Fund (CPF) has no elements of unemployment insurance." According to Ramesh (2004: 42):

> there is little state provision of income maintenance in Singapore, except for pensions for select government officials and public-assistance for the very poor. Provision, instead, takes the form of regulation of employers and employees to compulsorily save for retirement. The centerpiece in the income-maintenance system in Singapore is the CPF.

The CPF fund can be used for housing, old-age security, and hospitalization expenses. While it is a self-funded personal account of employed citizens, this is *not* to suggest that there is no state-provided benefit at all. Indeed, the state welfare budget increased after the Asian Financial Crisis, particularly through Community Development Councils and voluntary welfare organizations. At the moment, however, as Ramesh suggested, "they are discretionary payments that do not impose a long-term commitment on the government." In other words, the operating assumption is full employment, and welfare remains primarily each citizen's own responsibility.

Moreover, the emphasis of economic contribution can also be seen through how the state defines a "suitable" immigrant. First, according to the government report, *Population in Brief 2009* (National Population and Talent Division 2009):

> Singapore continues to face significant population challenges, brought about by persistently low fertility rates and, consequently, an ageing population. We will continue to adopt a three-prong approach of supporting more Singaporeans in getting married and having more children, facilitating the naturalization and integration of suitable foreigners, and engaging our overseas Singaporeans.

In answering a question from the audience concerning what constitutes a "suitable" immigrant at a university seminar, Mr. Tay Choon Hong, Director of Policy and Planning at the National Population and Talent Division in Singapore, said, "those who make economic contributions" (The Institute of Policy Studies 2011). More importantly, Singapore's foreign-worker policy is bifurcated, as shown

Table 1.5 Different eligibility schemes for employment pass and work permit holders

Type of pass	*Pass*	*Eligibility*	*Eligible for dependent pass?*	*Eligible for long term social visit pass?*
P	P1	For foreigners whose fixed monthly salary is more than S$7,000	Yes	Yes
	P2	For foreigners whose fixed monthly salary is more than S$3,500 and up to S$7,000	Yes	Yes
Q	Q1	For foreigners whose fixed monthly salary is more than S$2,500 and who possess acceptable degrees, professional qualifications or specialist skills	Yes	No
S	A new category of Work Pass which replaces the Q2 Pass with effect from July 1, 2004. The S Pass is for mid-skilled foreigners, whose fixed monthly salary is more than S$1,800		Yes (if monthly basic salary is equal or more than S$2,500)	No
WP	Work Permit issued to a skilled or an unskilled foreigner, who are from approved source country/territory, with a fixed monthly salary of not more than S$1,800 to work in Singapore		No	No

Source: Adapted from Ministry of Manpower (2011a).

in Table 1.5. At point of entry, higher-skilled and better-educated foreigners are given "employment passes," and low-skilled contract labor, "work permits." This two-tiered foreign-worker policy encourages the entry and settlement of skilled immigrants, while permitting the entry of unskilled workers but discouraging their settlement.

It is important to know not only the nature and character of a particular nation-state but also the context in which it has developed. Singapore became an independent nation abruptly in 1965, and immediately had to face the challenge of steering a viable economic course and the task of nation-building. One important strategy was export-led industrialization, involving the expansion of the manufacturing sector by multinational corporations. This, in turn, necessitated increasing the level of literacy in the population and, hence, significant social investment in education. The developmental state model intensified as Singapore transformed itself from a manufacturing-based economy to a knowledge-based economy by the late 1990s, particularly with regard to the service sector and higher-value-added industries related to biomedical sciences and digital media.

Chapter 3 contains a more detailed analysis of one of the channels through which productivism finds its expression via state welfare provision: the institutionalization of citizenship-as-responsibility primarily through the CPF and provision of state-subsidized housing. While this book concurs with Hill and Lian's (1995) claim that citizenship is primarily interpreted to confer "duties" by the Singapore state, it further raises the critical question of what it means to consider childbearing and childrearing in an environment where the state emphasizes citizens' responsibilities. Moreover, it should be noted not only that citizenship confers "duty," but that the state regards citizens as human resources.

The "human resources," not "human rights" paradigm

With regard to individuals who have citizenship status, the discourse of "human resources"—not "human rights"—predominates in Singapore. For example, Kwok and Ali (1998: 113) argued that "fundamentally . . . the people who constitute the [Singaporean] nation are regarded by the state as human resources." Osman-Gani (2004: 276) wrote:

> Human resources have been identified as the single most important strategic capital for Singapore. A small country with virtually no natural resources, Singapore has become one of the most developed countries in Asia primarily due to its strong emphasis on developing human resources and for continuously making significant investments in its human capital. Human resource development has always been a core element in its strategic economic plans.

More importantly, the economic success of Singapore has been significantly attributed to such a human resources paradigm (see also Akdere 2005; Quah 1998; Wan and Hui 2008; Yap 2009). How does the human-resource economic-development paradigm relate to theories of citizenship? I suggest that the state's emphasis on citizenship-as-responsibility connects seamlessly with the human-resource approach to economic development. That is, in the eyes of the state, citizens constitute the primary resources for the nation's economic growth, and citizens are mobilized on the premise that their well-being depends almost exclusively on their own or their family members' paid labor force participation.

Economic development and demographic transformation

While citizenship-as-responsibility and the developmental and productivist emphasis may have helped in Singapore's economic production, transformation, and rising geopolitical prominence, what do they mean for the nation-state's own social reproduction?

Among many policies formulated and implemented by the Singaporean government, one fundamental policy arena is population growth, not least because it concerns long-term management and mobilization of human resources for economic development. The state, through population policies, invests in the making of future citizens. Citizens, as parents and potential parents, also invest in future generations. Who is worthy of such investment, and what is considered necessary investment? State and citizens may not always agree.

Book outline

In subsequent chapters, I present and analyze findings based on in-depth individual and focus group interviews with 221 Singapore citizens concerning their perceptions and experiences in regard to pronatalist state policies. In Chapter 2, "Low fertility and pronatalist population policies," I begin with a review of studies on the phenomenon of below-replacement fertility in Europe and Asia, and identify two theoretical approaches underlying pronatalist policies: economic and institutional-cultural. The rest of the chapter situates Singapore's pronatalist policy initiatives since 2000 within these two broader theoretical approaches.

Chapter 3, "Economic development, social investments, and population control" substantiates one of the ways in which productivism is pursued—as Lee (2007: 15) suggested, "unlike Western welfare states where collective welfare is provided collectively, Singapore shuns the pooled risk system of social insurance and seeks to provide individualized welfare." I analyze the domestic institutions governing citizen-responsibility supporting Singapore's economic development, such as the People's Action Party's leadership, the structure of the educational system, and operations of the Central Provident Fund (CPF) and the Housing Development Board (HDB). Moreover, I locate Singapore's population control within the larger literature on population and economic development. Singapore has a more than half-century-long history of explicit state policies designed to control its population, and the rest of the chapter traces the continuity and change in such policies from anti- to pronatalist since independence in 1965.

Chapters 4 and 5 focus on the aspect of social reproduction, suggesting another route through which productivism expresses itself.

Chapter 4, "Class-differentiated pronatalism," focuses on the perception and effectiveness of economic incentives in Singapore's pronatalist policies. I argue that policy effectiveness is a function not only of the amount of economic support, but also of (1) the economic context in which incentives are perceived; (2) channels through which information concerning support is disseminated; and (3) forms in which financial incentives are distributed.

Chapter 5, "Privileging the citizen-worker," juxtaposes the gendered assumption of "citizen-workers" underlying pronatalist policies on work–family balance and the realities of citizens' varying relationships with work and family life. Interview data show heterogeneity among women and men in their preferences for a life centered on employment or the home, which necessarily entails differing responses and reactions toward such policies.

Chapter 6, "Constructing children's multi-dimensional qualities," highlights two perspectives (individual competitiveness versus interpersonal competence) and institutional factors (primarily the shift from a manufacturing to a knowledge-based economy) that contribute to limiting childbirth, particularly among respondents from middle-income households. Thus, while state policies aim at inducing parents to increase the number of children by providing an economic bonus, social class differences in decision making have generated a counterintuitive result for policies implemented since the mid-1980s.

Making future citizens

I argue that the gap between the stated aim of the pronatalist population policies and persistent low fertility reflects the limitations of the productivist paradigm, of which citizenship-as-responsibility is a key component. Moreover, I suggest that the state needs to recognize the growing importance of citizenship-as-social rights. First, there is a disjunction between the merit-based thrust of state policies and citizens' desires for a more supportive socio-economic environment as a precondition for having a child or additional child. While citizens who were interviewed as parents and prospective parents did not invoke individual rights, they did express desires for, in particular, state-provided or guaranteed access to education (or free education) and more subsidized healthcare and housing. Second, there is a mismatch between, on one hand, the state's assumption of "citizen-workers" and, on the other, parents and prospective parents' varying aspirations and social realities of "citizen-workers" and "citizen-parents." Third, encouraging childbirth among citizens is not solely a matter of providing economic resources or parental leave from work, but also construction of "ideal" citizens. If "individual competitiveness" reigns, particularly in the face of scarce resources, parents and prospective parents are likely to limit childbearing. Fourth, citizens have profound concerns about raising children with limited resources, and competing conceptions of quality in mind, which lead some citizens to consider migration to other countries that may offer a more supportive environment for parenting and child development (Sun 2010).

At the theoretical level, this study suggests the importance of contexts and of taking "bottom-up" constructs seriously in the field of citizenship studies. Research findings suggest that citizens' concerns about rising costs of living and job insecurity, and their perceptions of state subsidies benefiting particular groups (i.e., individuals with higher socio-economic status, career-oriented men, and family-oriented working women) have meant limited effectiveness of state policies in encouraging childbirth among the citizenry. There is a desire for the state to extend its range of direct provision from particular groups to all citizens, through universal financial subsidies, affordable education, healthcare, and housing provisions, as well as specific policies supporting work–family balance.

This study also suggests a reframing of debates on rights and responsibilities. The question is not whether citizen rights or responsibilities should be emphasized, but under what conditions, with what implications, and toward what goals? To the extent that citizens' desires for direct state financial subsidies are made in the context of global capitalism, rising income inequality, an increasing sense of job insecurity, and growing unequal access to education, this study suggests the importance of a context-dependent understanding of citizenship and demands on the state through the study of population policies.

Finally, this study suggests the importance of empirical engagement in social and public policy design. In particular, with regard to the debate surrounding whether there should be group-specific rights, with their attendant policy implications, this study suggests that the answer cannot be formed *a priori*. That is to say, what kinds of policies should be designed in relation to which specific groups requires empirical investigation. Part of the reason for this is that social group formation and identity are not fixed and static, and the notion of a minority group refers to relations of domination in a particular context rather than a statistical reality. For example, as far as pronatalist policies on work–family balance are concerned, the relevant identity issue seems to be citizen-worker or citizen-parent. Policies would have to be responsive to challenges that a particular group faces in order to be effective, and, in this case, if the goal is to facilitate social reproduction, the state needs to provide legal protection for rights to parenthood and paid employment. More generally, this book suggests that there needs to be greater social awareness in designing public policies. In other words, it is fruitful to see the relationship between state policies and individual behavior as, at least partly, a function of the knowledge, framing, interpretations, and understandings of such policies at the micro level. I consider the significance of these arguments in relation to the issue of migration in Chapter 7, the concluding chapter. I also sum up the analysis of data collected to answer questions on ethnic differentials in fertility rates in Singapore, and elaborate more fully on the productivist approach and inherent contradictions of the human-resource economic-development paradigm also adopted in other East Asian countries. The general proposition, I hope, facilitates more dialogue between state agencies and citizens with regard to their respective rights and responsibilities, and a more grounded understanding and articulation of multidimensional qualities of current and future citizens.

2 Low fertility and pronatalist population policies

In this chapter, we are concerned with the phenomenon of below replacement-level fertility, consequences typically associated with it, and two common types of state pronatalist population policies—financial incentives and work–family-balance policies—designed to encourage citizens to have more children.

Global trends in fertility behavior

Fertility declined worldwide in the second half of the twentieth century, particularly among industrializing and newly industrialized countries. During this period, post-industrial European countries were experiencing the second demographic transition (Lesthaeghe 1995; van de Kaa 1987), characterized by declining marriage rates, below-replacement fertility rates, rising ages at first marriage and childbearing, and increasing cohabitation, divorce, and non-marital fertility. In East and Southeast Asia, the decline in birth rates during the same period was even more dramatic; Gubhaju and Moriki-Durand (2003: 1) succinctly described that "the total fertility rate (TFR) of around six children per woman in the period 1950–1955 dropped by more than half to 2.7 in the period 1995–2000." Moreover, as shown in Table 2.1, several newly industrialized countries of Asia have entered an era of below-replacement fertility.[1] Indeed, according to Jones *et al.* (2009: 1):

> a new problem is emerging, with its key locus in Pacific Asia . . . This problem is ultra-low fertility. Japan, Singapore, Taiwan, South Korea, and Hong Kong SAR are among the very lowest-fertility countries in the whole world, and even China has reached fertility levels lower than those in many European countries.

Kohler *et al.* (2002) coined the term "lowest-low fertility" for a period TFR below 1.3. Dire consequences associated with below-replacement fertility and lowest-low fertility have been highlighted in the literature and official reports, prominent among these are population decline, population aging, labor shortages and increasing elderly dependency ratios, as well as increased dependence on immigration, which, in turn, generates rising conflicts between citizens and non-citizens.

First, with respect to the issue of population decline, country-specific years for the beginning of population decline in certain Asian countries, as projected by the

Table 2.1 Trends in total fertility rates and projected population growth, selected East Asian countries

Total fertility rate	*Japan*	*South Korea*	*Taiwan*	*Singapore*	*Hong Kong SAR*
1995	1.42	1.64	1.78	1.67	n.a.
1996	1.43	1.70	1.76	1.66	1.19
1997	1.39	1.54	1.77	1.61	1.12
1998	1.38	1.47	1.47	1.47	1.02
1999	1.34	1.42	1.56	1.47	0.98
2000	1.36	1.47	1.68	1.60	1.04
2001	1.33	1.30	1.40	1.41	0.93
2002	1.32	1.17	1.34	1.37	0.94
2003	1.29	1.17	1.24	1.25	0.90
2004	1.29	1.16	1.18	1.24	0.93
2005	1.25	1.08	1.12	1.25	0.97
2006	1.32	1.13	1.12	1.26	0.98
2007	1.30	1.30	1.12	1.30	1.00
2008	1.40	1.20	1.00	1.30	1.10
2009	1.40	1.30	n.a.	1.20	1.00
Projected % growth, UN medium projection, 2005–2030					
Population	–4.3	2.8		20.2	22.3
15–64 age group	–17.0	–8.7		–0.3	4.2
15–24 age group	–20.0	–36.9		–25.2	–15.3
Projected % growth, UN low projection, 2005–2030					
Population	–9.9	–4.3		12.7	13.0
15–64 age group	–19.8	–12.2		–3.3	0.9
15–24 age group	–37.7	–53.1		–42.3	–38.2

Source: Adapted from Jones *et al.* (2009); World Bank (2011).

United Nations' *World Population Prospects: The 2010 Revision*, are as follows: Japan after 2010, South Korea after 2030, Taiwan after 2015, and Singapore after 2040 (United Nations 2010).

Second, with respect to population aging, according to the report *Asia's Aging Population*, "the process of population aging [in Asia] is occurring much more rapidly than it did in Western countries, and it will occur in some Asian countries at a much earlier stage of economic development" (East-West Center 2008: 83). Chan (2005: 271) suggested that "by the year 2030, the two oldest Asian countries will be Singapore and Japan." Indeed, according to *World Population Prospects: The 2008 Revision* (the latest data for which estimates are available), Japan can expect 30.8 percent of its population to be aged 65 and above in the year 2030, whereas Singapore and South Korea will have at least 27.5 percent and 23.2 percent, respectively, of their populations at or above the age of 65 by the same year.

Third, regarding the issue of labor shortage, Gubhaju and Moriki-Durand (2003: 7) portray the possible development of a shrinking working-age population in Asia:

> Changes in the age structure of the population are more pronounced in countries where fertility declined rapidly. Japan will experience a considerable drop in the proportion of the working-age population—by the year 2050, it will be only a little over half the population. Korea and Singapore will also have decreased proportions in the working ages (56 and 57 per cent respectively) in 2050.

The old age dependency ratio (defined as the number of persons aged 65 and over per working person aged 15–64) for Japan, South Korea, and Singapore are projected to increase from 25, 10, and 10 in 2000, respectively, to 72, 55, and 54 in 2050 (United Nations 2002). Increases in old age dependency ratios reflect that fewer working age persons will be available to support older persons in the future.

Fourth, at present, Europe's population is increasing, due to immigration. Reflecting a similar trend, the fertility rate in the United States hit 2.1 in 2006 for the first time in 35 years (Hamilton, Martin, and Ventura 2007). Caldwell and Schindlmayr (2003: 243) made the observation that this "higher fertility is partly a reflection of immigrant Hispanic reproductive behaviour." Massive immigration, however, breeds resentment and prejudice, even though laws in most countries ban discrimination against foreigners. As Newman described it:

> In Great Britain, the antipathy is directed against immigrants from India and Pakistan; in France, against Algerians and Moroccans; in Germany, Turks; in Sweden, Iraqis and Kurds; in Australia, South and East Asians; in the United States, immigrants from Latin America and Asia; and in Japan, almost anyone not Japanese.
>
> (2004: 482)

Thus, despite the economic necessity of immigrant labor, many industrialized countries have exercised strict control of immigration. Moreover, according to McDonald (2002: 2), "where fertility is below 1.6, the levels of migration required for replacement of the population become impossibly large." In Asia, Singapore currently has the highest proportion of immigrants and, in 2006 (the latest data for which detailed statistics of employment by citizenship status are available), approximately 30 percent of its paid labor force were foreigners (60 percent were Singapore citizens and 10 percent were permanent residents). As elsewhere, in light of growing tensions between locals and immigrants, "the government has reduced the annual intake of migrant workers from 150,000 to 100,000; it has also raised levies on foreign workers to make it less attractive for companies to import labor" (Oi 2010).

In short, in light of potential problems such as population decline, population aging, a shrinking workforce, and rising social conflicts, governments in advanced industrialized countries in Europe and Asia have launched initiatives to encourage more births among citizens. Among the 30 countries in the Organization for Economic Cooperation and Development (OECD) that reported to the United Nations on policies designed to maintain or raise fertility levels, only seven reported that they had such policies in place in 1996. However, that number had risen to 13 by 2003; and more countries have announced pronatalist policies since then (d'Addio and d'Ercole 2005: 47). Even in China, the TFR "has truly fallen below the replacement level of 2.1 [since 2000]" and has "definitely reached the stage of low fertility" (Gu 2009: 75). The Chinese government is considering a gradual shift away from its one-child policy in light of an aging population, although it plans to keep the current policy for another decade (Yardley 2008).

In surveying the literature on state pronatalist policies, I highlight two kinds of government policies:

1. provision of financial incentives, and
2. work–family-balance policies.

The economic approach and financial incentives

Insofar as pronatalist *financial* benefits are concerned, governments in different countries have implemented a variety of measures, ranging from cash bonuses to various tax relief schemes. Below, I provide a brief review of empirical studies on the effectiveness of such financial measures. First, in terms of cash subsidies, Cigno and Ermisch (1989) found that higher child benefits increased British women's completed fertility. Using an econometric model for data from 22 industrialized countries from 1970 to 1990, Gauthier and Hatzius (1997: 304) found cash benefits to be positively correlated to fertility; specifically:

> a 25 per cent increase in family allowances would result in a fertility level which is about 0.6 per cent higher in the short-run and about 4 per cent higher in the long-run—that is, an effect on the order of 0.07 children per woman on average.

Neyer (2003) reviewed studies on family policies' effects on fertility among low-fertility countries in Western Europe and noted that:

> By 1985 most countries with previously employment-based child-benefit systems had switched to universal cash benefits, and, in the majority of these countries (7 out of 13), the mother received the benefit. In addition, between the 1950s and the 1980s almost all countries amended their systems to make families eligible for child benefits independent of the number of children, the family income, or the family status. As a consequence, in 2001 only five Western European countries tie the claim to child benefits to employment or employment-based insurance, namely the Southern European countries and Belgium.

As Neyer (2003) put it, "child benefits are thus the family-policy measure that is most widely governed by the principle of social rights." In Sweden, Bjorklund (2006: 3) examined family policies that offered financial and in-kind support to families for childbirth and found that "the extension of the policy raised the level of fertility, shortened the spacing of births and induced fluctuations in the period fertility rates." Studies of the birth bonus in the province of Quebec, in Canada, also suggest a positive impact on fertility—although, again, at a rather high cost per child. Kim (2007) noted that the Allowance for Newborn Children (ANC) cost more than C$19,000 for one extra birth, which was higher than an earlier estimate of C$15,000 (Milligan 2002).

With regard to pronatalist financial incentives in terms of tax breaks, Whittington, Alm and Peter (1990) found that personal tax exemptions had a positive and significant effect on the national birth rate in the United States, and suggested that it would be possible to influence citizens' fertility decisions to some degree through deliberate changes in tax policies. However, Georgellis and Wall (1992) examined the US tax exemption scheme and found that tax exemption as a form of subsidy for childbearing increased fertility but its effect was very limited.

In sum, most empirical studies seem to suggest that pronatalist financial subsidies have a positive effect on fertility rates. However, as Gauthier's (2007) review pointed out, such impact on fertility trends tended to be limited and varied highly according to type of policy and type of data used. Moreover, recent studies conducted in Central and Eastern Europe pointed to the critical importance of the stability of financial support and the status of the overall economy in shaping effectiveness of pronatalist financial measures (Rostgaard 2004; Saxonberg and Szelewa 2007; Stewart and Huerta 2006).

The institutional–cultural approach and work–family-balance policies

As Yamaguchi and Lee (2008: 7) put it, "generally, we can expect that the relationship between female labor-force participation and fertility rate is not uniform but varies with the extent to which work–family balance can be attained and thereby reduce the opportunity costs of childrearing." Recent studies have looked into different forms of state pronatalist policies supporting work–family balance—including, but not limited to, maternity and paternity leave and accessibility of childcare services—and their impact on individual childbearing behavior. For example, Letablier (2003) examined French family policy, which shifted its objective from supporting direct costs of having children to supporting work–family reconciliation, and concluded that policies that help support individuals reconcile the conflicting demands of work and family have helped to keep fertility rates at an acceptable level. In terms of maternity leave policies, Ronsen (2004) investigated determinants of the fertility process in Finland and Norway, and found that extension of maternity leave had a positive impact on fertility, especially for higher-order births. Similarly, Risse (2006) found that availability of maternity leave elevated the likelihood of pregnancy in Australia, although this effect depended on a woman's age and whether the maternity leave was paid or unpaid.

In terms of accessibility of childcare services and places, Castles' (2003) study examining data from 21 OECD countries contains two important findings. First, the ability of women to access childcare places they need and to arrange their lives in ways that can accommodate work and family conflicts is crucial to positive fertility outcomes. Second, fertility outcome is a function of education and labor-market policies that enhance the probability of women finding employment irrespective of their fertility behavior. This second finding suggests that assuring women of secured jobs could be the key to positive fertility outcomes. Similarly, Bonoli (2008) found that, in Switzerland, childcare availability and generosity of child benefits had a positive impact on fertility; she suggested that a positive effect on fertility could be achieved by meeting demands of women and families in terms of reconciling work and family life.

Perhaps more importantly, it is not just work–family-balance policies that are important but also the "gendered" context in which such policies take effect. McDonald (2000: 427) suggested that "very low fertility in advanced countries today is an outcome of a conflict or inconsistency between high levels of gender equity in individual-oriented social institutions and sustained gender inequity in family-oriented social institutions." Olah (2003: 193) found that "couples who share family responsibilities more equally have higher second-birth intensity than others when policies facilitate the combination of employment and parenting for either parent." In other words, low fertility is driven by the discrepancy between gender equality in the public sphere and gender inequality in the domestic sphere.

While Olah's and McDonald's frameworks treated men and women as constituting homogeneous groups, Hakim (2003: 369–70) presented findings from a national survey in Britain and proposed that the development of family and population policy needs to start with the recognition that women and men differ in their values, goals, and aspirations:

> The current emphasis on the first and second demographic transitions overlooks the fundamental importance of the recent sea change in fertility control. When women control their own fertility, it is their preferences and values that shape responses to public policy. And public policy has not, in practice, paid much attention to women's wishes . . . It is this heterogeneity of lifestyle preferences [of a life centered on employment or other competitive activities in the public sphere or else a life centered on the noncompetitive activities of private life] that impedes attempts to predict fertility.

In line with Hakim's preference theory, Shkolnikov *et al.* (2007) statistically analyzed the growing concentration of reproduction in cohorts of women in Europe and the United States. Fertility behavior was found to vary across women. Shkolnikov *et al.* (2007: 92) thus suggested that "future family policies should not simply focus on 'average' women or 'average working mothers' but should also address a spectrum of orientations and life strategies." Sweden stands out as a case in which population policies respect and recognize heterogeneity in the life plans of citizens. In his review of research on the role that social and family policies play in fertility in Sweden, Andersson (2008: 90) wrote:

> It is important to note that Swedish family policy has never specifically targeted childbearing but has rather aimed at strengthening women's participation in the labor market and promoting gender and social equality. The focus has been on enabling individuals to pursue their family and occupational tracks without being too dependent on other persons or being constrained by institutional factors. In terms of childbearing, the goal is to enable women and men to raise the number of children they want to have.

The history of Swedish innovative programs is also instructive, as it highlights the shifting policy focus from women to men:

> In the 1970s and 1980s, changes in women's position in society motivated the introduction of a wide range of policies with the aim of achieving greater compatibility between women's role in the family and at work. Subsequently, public policies have continued to aim at promoting gender equality but then focused more explicitly on men and their reconciliation of family and work.
>
> (Andersson 2008: 90)

Along similar lines, Neyer's review of the effects of family polices on fertility in low-fertility countries in Western Europe also broadly concluded that:

> Countries which regard these [pronatalist] policies as parts of labor-market policies, of care policies, and of gender policies seem to have fared better in retaining fertility above the labor market so that both *women and men* are able to maintain employment and income, even if they have (small) children to care for. (my emphasis)
>
> (2003: 69)

Although citizens' responses toward state work–family-balance policies are the central concern of this book, studies investigating perceptions and responses toward such policies offered by companies are instructive. For example, employees with relatively more privilege are more likely to have access to but less likely to make use of work–life benefits or flexible arrangements. Wharton, Chivers, and Blair-Loy (2008: 327) suggested that:

> consistent with the work devotion perspective, it was found that formal work-family policies are more widely used among hourly workers than managers, and those with better performance evaluations are less likely than their otherwise similar co-workers to use formal work–family policies.

Their studies reflected the problem of how employees were appraised and how their devotion and commitment were measured. As Blair-Loy and Wharton (2004: 260) noted:

> employees reporting no interest [in the work–family-balance policies] are in the minority, yet they are among the most senior and most highly paid . . . They

> put in the longest hours . . . Many have family situations that offer little competition to their work, as they are significantly more likely than other groups to have a homemaking spouse.

These studies suggest that working women may be subject to the same structural constraints as men in terms of the standardized measurement of work devotion and potential wage penalty entailed in taking time off for care giving.

Male workers who are interested in increasing family time may find even more obstacles than their female counterparts. Cunningham (2001), for example, illustrated the gendered assumption in family-friendly policy in law firms: While women can take childcare paid leave, male attorneys must meet "primary caregiver" criteria in order to enjoy the same benefits. Even in Sweden, where companies are more father-friendly (giving extensive "daddy days," parental leave for male employees), men's use of state-mandated family leave benefits remains modest, as wider changes in corporate policy and practice are ignored (Haas and Hwang 1995). For example, fathers report that employers, supervisors, and male co-workers do not look favorably on their interest in taking parental leave.

Boling (2008) provided additional insights into causes of the prolonged and sharp fall in total fertility in Japan through comparing the case of Japan to that of France. She reminded us that one needs to understand the work culture and labor market structure contexts in which work–family-balance policies take effect:

> Although significant, the gap between French and Japanese family-friendly policies does not alone explain the differences in TFRs in the two countries. Crucial to understanding Japan's low fertility is the fact that Japan is a "long hours" work culture where families and working parents are under greater pressures than their French counterparts.
>
> (p. 312)

In summary, our understanding of the effectiveness of work–family-balance policies has been furthered by the above-mentioned research conducted in advanced industrialized countries. Taken together, the studies suggest that there is a need to analyze policy effectiveness in relation to possible differences in priority that individual women and men place on family and on paid employment. Moreover, it is important to pay attention to local work cultures. In the next section, I provide a succinct review of studies on the topic of pronatalist policies' impacts [in Asia] before elaborating on Singapore's state pronatalist incentives.

The impact of pronatalist policies on fertility in Asian countries

As Jones *et al.* (2009: 15) pointed out in their review of pronatalist policies on fertility in Asian countries, "the general consensus about pronatalist policies in East Asian countries seems to be that they have failed, because there is no evidence that fertility has risen as a result of their introduction." For instance, McDonald and

Evans (2002: 10) noted "the failure of substantial direct financial incentives in various levels and forms to influence the fertility level of Singapore Chinese," arguing that "incentives in the form of reduced opportunity costs of having children will be more effective than incentives in the form of cash subsidies." At the same time, studies have indicated a slowly emerging heterogeneity in women's relationship with paid employment and the family. For example, Ogawa, Retherford, and Matsukura (2006: 66–67) suggested that in order to improve pronatalist policy effectiveness in Japan, "it is useful to consider the effects of these [pronatalist] programs on two groups of women: those who work for pay outside the home and those who do not work for pay outside the home."

Employed women in advanced Asian countries certainly experienced stress in juggling work and home responsibilities. In the case of South Korea, Choe (2006) highlighted the increasing trend of women entering career-oriented jobs and that the majority of nonworking married women would prefer to be employed, if not for the problem of childcare. Quah (2009: 116) documented that women in Hong Kong and Singapore find work and family responsibilities irreconcilable without men sharing family responsibilities:

> Hong Kong and particularly Singapore women join the labor force in large proportions in their twenties but their resolve to tackle both home and job commitments falters and they begin withdrawing steadily from the labor force after marriage or after the arrival of their first child due to the burden of family obligations.

More importantly, Quah emphasized that

> the higher status given to the husband as the principal economic provider has not changed much in the past three decades, at least not in Asia although working women's earnings in the wealthier countries—Japan, Hong Kong and Singapore—are increasing.
>
> (2009: 127)

Thus, Quah (2009: 128) suggested that "the main challenge for sociologists studying gender roles is to identify through further research the best possible avenues for both men and women to be able to attain their life and family goals at minimum cost and optimum gain."

Low fertility and pronatalist incentives in Singapore

As alluded to in Chapter 1 and illustrated below in Figure 2.1, fertility in Singapore fell in 1977 and has remained below replacement level ever since.

The earlier "Girl or Boy, Two Is Enough" anti-natalist policy of the 1960s and 1970s officially gave way to pronatalist policies in 1987. During the transition period, the political leadership was concerned not only about increasing the national birth rate to replacement level, but doing so specifically among the higher-educated

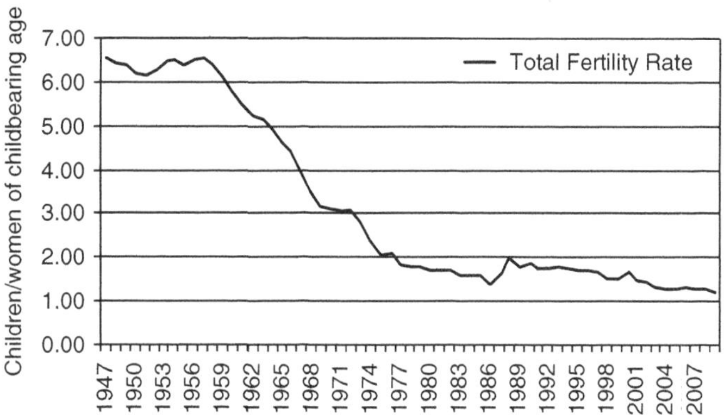

Figure 2.1 Total fertility rates (TFR), Singapore, 1947–2009

Sources: Saw (1980); Singapore Department of Statistics (2009a, 2010a).

sector of the population. Hence the "Graduate-Mother Priority Scheme," based on then Prime Minister Lee Kuan Yew's 1983 National Day speech on the need for redressing the "lopsided" pattern of lower fertility among women with tertiary education, failing which, he warned:

> Levels of competence will decline. Our economy will falter, the administration will suffer, and the society decline. For how can we avoid lowering performance when for every two graduates, in 25 years' time there will be one graduate, and for every two uneducated workers, there will be three?
>
> (Cited in Saw 1990: 43)

Earlier studies of pronatalist policies highlighted a concern with eugenics and class-based differentiation (Drakakis-Smith and Graham 1996; Palen 1986; Wee, 1995). For example, in analyzing the thrust of the 1983 speech, Wee characterized the historical shift as changing from a "universally applicable" approach to "a differential class-specific pronatalism" (1995: 201). Indeed, the Graduate-Mother Priority Scheme, introduced in 1984, offered priority in primary school registration for children of women with university degrees or professionals, a move that generated popular resentment. In 1984 the People's Action Party (PAP) suffered significant election losses. In 1985 the scheme was discontinued.

Since then, there has been no clear and overt educational bias in pronatalist incentives. As Palen (1986: 3) noted:

> the initial eugenics-based program introduced in 1984 sought increased fertility for university-educated women and provided major subsidies for the voluntary sterilization of poor and uneducated parents. These much publicized and internationally discussed programs have now been abandoned in favor of new population programs seeking to encourage fertility in lower as well as better educated groups. A 40 per cent population increase is being set as a goal.

In 1987 the government launched policy incentives under the theme "Have Three, or More If You Can Afford It." Emphasis was now placed on the adequacy of economic resources rather than parents' educational qualifications. Drakakis-Smith and Graham (1996: 69) examined the views of Singaporeans towards such policy measures based on a representative survey carried out in 1992. The authors concluded that:

> although differences in fertility behaviour may be rooted in ethnic identity, the control that the government wishes to exert over that behaviour as part of its nation-building project has largely been effected through class interests [measured as monthly household income].

In recent years, further policy amendments have been implemented, with incentives growing wider in scope and more elaborate, aiming at "bringing Singapore's population growth back to the replacement level of 2.1 children per woman" (Ministry of Education, Singapore 2007). In 2000 the policy theme was "Strong and Stable Families," and, in 2004, the slogan was changed to "Singapore. A Great Place For Families." Monetary incentives were organized primarily via taxation, while non-monetary incentives included housing, education, and employment, among others (Lin and Rantalaiho 2003). The government's proposed expenditure on pronatalist policy initiatives increased dramatically from S$500 million in 2001, to S$800 million in 2004, then to S$1600 million in 2008 (National Population and Talent Division 2011a).

I identify seven pronatalist policy initiatives that can be categorized under the economic approach to raising fertility that were in force when this study was carried out: income tax relief, tax rebates, childcare subsidies, use of Medisave accounts (i.e., savings in the medical savings account of provident fund savings), maid levy subsidies, cash benefits, and grandparent caregiver tax relief. The first five policy incentives (ranging from income tax relief to maid levy subsidies) have been in existence in some form since 1987. The government instituted two additional economic initiatives (cash benefits and grandparent caregiver relief) in 2000. Details of the pronatalist policies and their historical changes between 1987 and 2008 can be seen in Appendix A. In what follows, I provide a brief summary of pronatalist benefits as of August 2008:

1. Income tax relief: Tax relief was increased to S$4,000 per child for all children in 2008. In addition, percentages of tax relief claimable for each child have been increased, varying between 15 and 25 percent. The maximum claimable vis-à-vis working mothers' earned income has also increased to S$50,000.
2. Tax rebates: The S$20,000 tax rebate for a third child in 1987 was extended to a fourth child in 1989. Moreover, the S$10,000 tax rebate was set conditionally for a second child in 2000. In 2008, the tax rebate was further extended, the first child was granted a S$5,000 rebate, and the fifth child and beyond was also granted the S$20,000 rebate.

3. Childcare subsidies: For working mothers, the monthly infant-care (2–18 months) subsidy was increased to S$600 and the monthly childcare (19 months to 7 years) subsidy was increased to S$300 in 2008. For nonworking mothers, both infant-care and childcare monthly subsidies were increased to S$150.
4. Use of Medisave account: In 1987, parents were allowed to use their savings in medical savings accounts (of the Central Provident Fund savings) for delivery and hospitalization charges for a third child; this usage was extended to a fourth child in 2004, and further extended to the first four children in 2008. Since 2004 this account has also been permitted to be used for assisted conception procedures.
5. Maid levy subsidies: There was maid levy tax relief for working mothers in 1987; the amount of this monthly levy was reduced from S$345 to S$250 in 2004, and further reduced to S$170 in 2008.
6. Cash benefits: Cash benefits are arguably the most recent and proactive form of economic incentives. In April 2000 the government started the "Baby Bonus" Scheme. This scheme consists of a two-tier payment given annually by the government for six years after the birth of a child. The first tier is a cash gift, and the second resembles a co-savings arrangement whereby the government matches dollar-for-dollar the annual amount the parents put into the child's Children Development Account. In April 2004 and August 2008, the baby bonus scheme was extended. The cash gift that parents receive now amounts to S$4,000 each for first and second children, and S$6,000 each for third and fourth children. There is, however, no cash benefit for a fifth child and beyond. The co-savings arrangement enables parents to receive a maximum of S$6,000 for their first and second child. Matching for third and fourth children is capped at S$12,000. For a fifth child and beyond, government contributions are up to S$18,000.
7. Grandparent caregiver tax relief: Since 2004, working mothers have been able to claim tax relief of S$3,000 if their parents or parents-in-law look after their children younger than 12 years old. This relief remained unchanged in 2008.

The government has also offered a range of non-monetary incentives since 1987 to encourage childbirth, as Appendix A indicates. For instance, five "work–life support" pronatalist policy initiatives were in place when the present study was carried out:

1. The flexible work arrangement for civil servants: The flexible hours scheme was instituted in 2000, and there was a shift from a five-and-a-half-day workweek to a five-day workweek in the civil service in 2004. The total number of hours for every employee remained at 42 per week.
2. Public sector leave: Childcare leave and conditional sterilization leave had been granted for female civil servants since 1987. Government employees were permitted to take three days' paid marriage leave upon getting married for the first time in 2000, the same year that fathers in the civil service were permitted to take three days' paternity leave for their first three children.

3. Extra paid maternity leave: The leave period was lengthened from 8 weeks in 2000 to 12 weeks for the first four births in 2004, and four weeks' maternity leave was established for adoptions.
4. Paid childcare leave: In 2004, two days of employer-paid statutory childcare leave were introduced for each working parent with children under the age of seven.
5. The "Work-Life Works!" fund: In 2004, a S$10 million fund was set up, and all private sector organizations became eligible to apply for grants from the fund to defray the cost of introducing measures to help employees better achieve work–life harmony.

The most recent changes in pronatalist policies supporting work–life balance were introduced in August 2008. These include the following:

1. Paid maternity leave was extended from 12 to 16 weeks. The last eight weeks of leave may be taken flexibly over a period of 12 months with mutual agreement between employer and employee.
2. Maternity leave protection was introduced, such that employers are required to pay maternity leave benefits if a woman is dismissed without sufficient cause within six months before the birth of a child or retrenched within the last three months of pregnancy.
3. Paid childcare leave was extended from two to six days per year.
4. Six days' unpaid infant care leave was introduced.

The government disseminated information via user-friendly brochures illustrated in cartoon style, which are also available online.[2] Major TV news channels and daily newspapers also covered the topic of pronatalist policies and childbearing on a daily and weekly basis, particularly during the first year after the policy took effect.

Existing studies on Singapore's pronatalist population policies

Anderson (2004), Saw (2007), and Wong and Yeoh (2003) have provided comprehensive overviews of fertility policies. Specifically, Wong and Yeoh (2003: 17–19) conducted content analysis of pronatalist population policies implemented in 2000, and suggested that such policies promote fertility within the "normal" family of married couples and government rhetoric "strongly implicate the woman by linking her to the area of reproduction." Anderson (2004) discussed in detail the changes in Singapore's population policies to suggest that this is "policy overshoots its original goal." *The Population of Singapore* (Saw 2007), similar to its predecessors, provided authoritative details of the policies and a description of Singapore's switch from anti-natalism to pronatalism.

Other recent studies on Singapore's fertility policies have suggested the importance of generational differences and macro-level economic situations in influencing individual fertility behavior. For example, Graham, Teo, Yeoh, and Levy (2002:

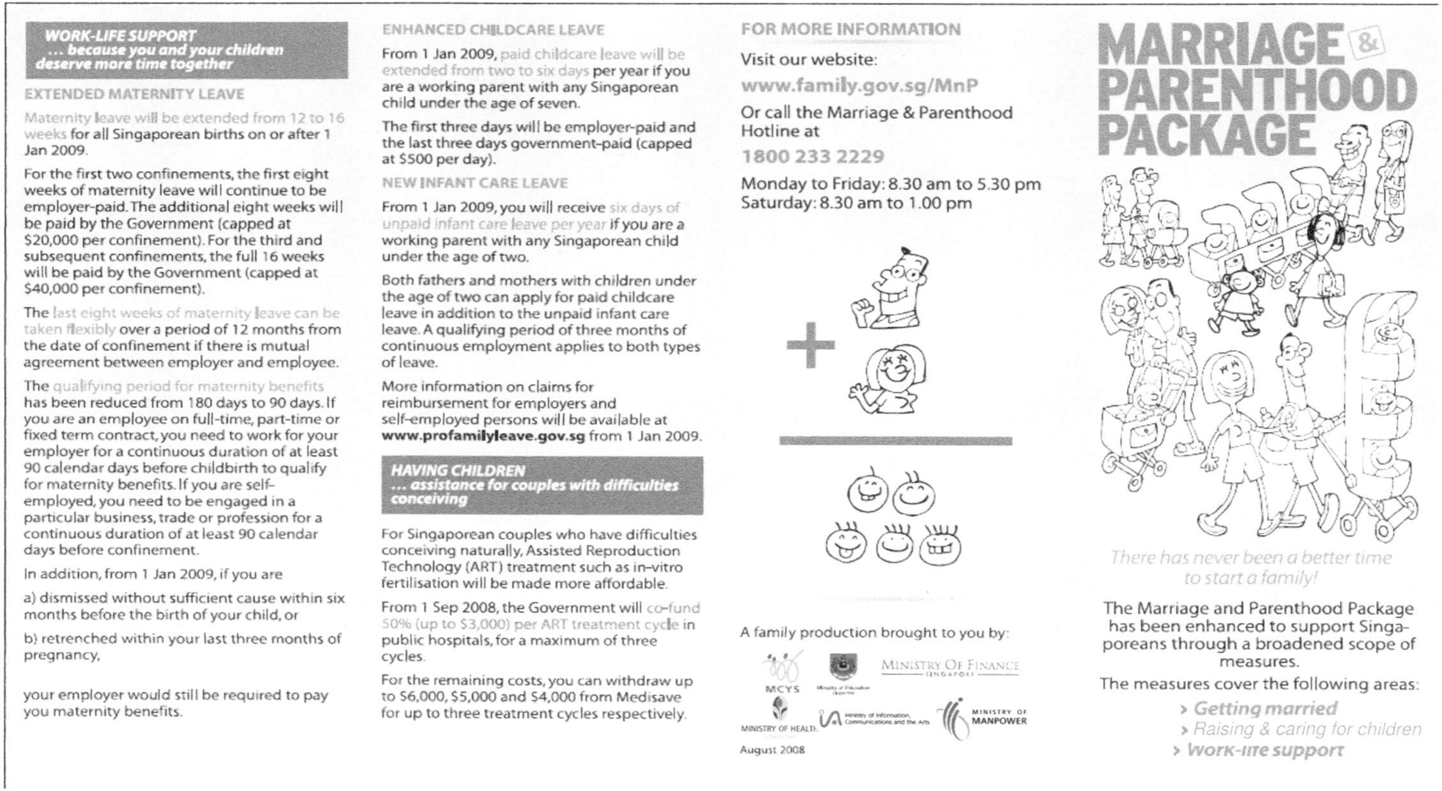

WORK-LIFE SUPPORT
... because you and your children deserve more time together

EXTENDED MATERNITY LEAVE

Maternity leave will be extended from 12 to 16 weeks for all Singaporean births on or after 1 Jan 2009.

For the first two confinements, the first eight weeks of maternity leave will continue to be employer-paid. The additional eight weeks will be paid by the Government (capped at $20,000 per confinement). For the third and subsequent confinements, the full 16 weeks will be paid by the Government (capped at $40,000 per confinement).

The last eight weeks of maternity leave can be taken flexibly over a period of 12 months from the date of confinement if there is mutual agreement between employer and employee.

The qualifying period for maternity benefits has been reduced from 180 days to 90 days. If you are an employee on full-time, part-time or fixed term contract, you need to work for your employer for a continuous duration of at least 90 calendar days before childbirth to qualify for maternity benefits. If you are self-employed, you need to be engaged in a particular business, trade or profession for a continuous duration of at least 90 calendar days before confinement.

In addition, from 1 Jan 2009, if you are

a) dismissed without sufficient cause within six months before the birth of your child, or

b) retrenched within your last three months of pregnancy,

your employer would still be required to pay you maternity benefits.

ENHANCED CHILDCARE LEAVE

From 1 Jan 2009, paid childcare leave will be extended from two to six days per year if you are a working parent with any Singaporean child under the age of seven.

The first three days will be employer-paid and the last three days government-paid (capped at $500 per day).

NEW INFANT CARE LEAVE

From 1 Jan 2009, you will receive six days of unpaid infant care leave per year if you are a working parent with any Singaporean child under the age of two.

Both fathers and mothers with children under the age of two can apply for paid childcare leave in addition to the unpaid infant care leave. A qualifying period of three months of continuous employment applies to both types of leave.

More information on claims for reimbursement for employers and self-employed persons will be available at **www.profamilyleave.gov.sg** from 1 Jan 2009.

HAVING CHILDREN
... assistance for couples with difficulties conceiving

For Singaporean couples who have difficulties conceiving naturally, Assisted Reproduction Technology (ART) treatment such as in-vitro fertilisation will be made more affordable.

From 1 Sep 2008, the Government will co-fund 50% (up to $3,000) per ART treatment cycle in public hospitals, for a maximum of three cycles.

For the remaining costs, you can withdraw up to $6,000, $5,000 and $4,000 from Medisave for up to three treatment cycles respectively.

FOR MORE INFORMATION

Visit our website:

www.family.gov.sg/MnP

Or call the Marriage & Parenthood Hotline at

1800 233 2229

Monday to Friday: 8.30 am to 5.30 pm
Saturday: 8.30 am to 1.00 pm

A family production brought to you by:

MCYS · Ministry of Finance Singapore · Ministry of Health · Ministry of Information, Communications and the Arts · Ministry of Manpower

August 2008

MARRIAGE & PARENTHOOD PACKAGE

There has never been a better time to start a family!

The Marriage and Parenthood Package has been enhanced to support Singaporeans through a broadened scope of measures.

The measures cover the following areas:

› Getting married
› Raising & caring for children
› Work-life support

Figure 2.2 Marriage parenthood package pamphlet

GETTING MARRIED...
... or looking for that special someone?

The Social Development Unit (SDU) and the Social Development Service (SdS) will be merged to offer more opportunities for singles to interact through a network of contacts while developing private dating agencies through accreditation.

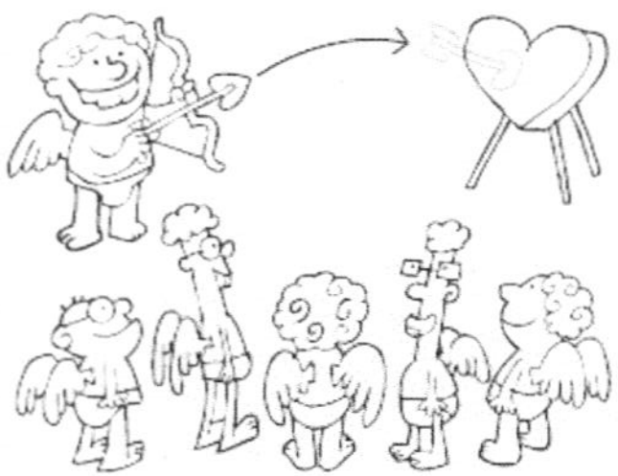

RAISING AND CARING FOR CHILDREN...
...can be made easier with some support

ENHANCED TAX BENEFITS

The Parenthood Tax Rebate (PTR) will be extended to all qualifying Singaporean children who are born or legally adopted on or after 1 Jan 2008.

Child order	Existing	Enhanced
First	-	**$5,000**
Second	$10,000	$10,000
Third & fourth	$20,000 for each child	**$20,000** for each child
Fifth & beyond	-	

Both father and mother may share the PTR to offset the income tax payable. Any unutilised rebate can be used to offset the income tax payable for subsequent years.

The Qualifying Child Relief (QCR) has increased from $2,000 to $4,000 per child and the Handicapped Child Relief (HCR) from $3,500 to $5,500 per child.

A working mother with Singaporean children will also enjoy the enhanced Working Mother's Child Relief (WMCR) up to 100% for all her qualifying children.

Child order	Existing	Enhanced % of mother's earned income
First	5%	**15%**
Second	15%	**20%**
Third	20%	**25%** for each child
Fourth	25%	
Fifth & beyond	-	

The total amount of QCR/HCR and WMCR claimable for each child is capped at $50,000.

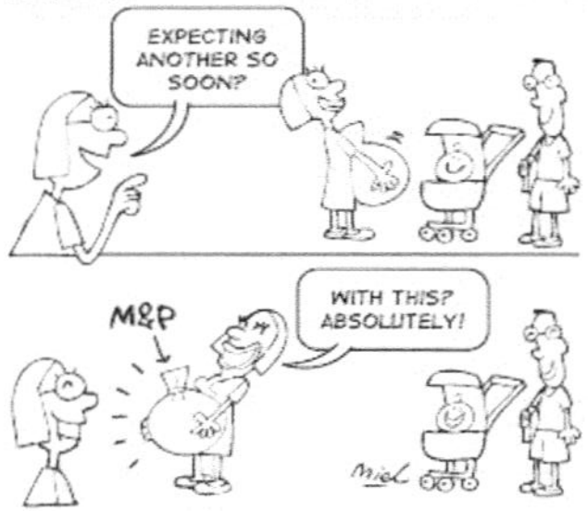
EXPECTING ANOTHER SO SOON?
M&P
WITH THIS? ABSOLUTELY!
Miel

ENHANCED BABY BONUS

The Baby Bonus cash gift and matching government contribution through the Children Development Account (CDA) have been enhanced for Singaporean babies born on or after 1 Jan 2009 to lawfully married parents.

Baby Bonus cash gift

Child order	Existing for each child	Enhanced for each child
First & second	$3,000	**$4,000**
Third & fourth	$6,000	$6,000

Baby Bonus CDA

Child order	Existing	Enhanced
First	-	**$6,000**
Second	$6,000	$6,000
Third & fourth	$12,000	$12,000
Fifth & beyond	-	**$18,000** for each child

The cash gift is given out in four equal instalments over 18 months. The Government will match dollar-for-dollar the amount of savings you contribute to your child's CDA up to the specified ceiling.

ENHANCED CENTRE-BASED CARE

More childcare centres will be set up over the next five years to provide more quality and affordable childcare options for working parents.

The quality of childcare services will be raised through higher educational and qualification requirements for pre-school teachers. Scholarships will be awarded to deserving pre-school teachers in childcare centres.

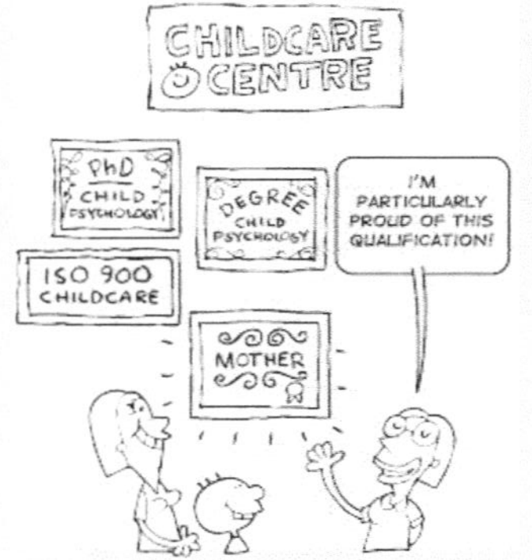
CHILDCARE CENTRE
PhD CHILD PSYCHOLOGY
DEGREE CHILD PSYCHOLOGY
ISO 900 CHILDCARE
MOTHER
I'M PARTICULARLY PROUD OF THIS QUALIFICATION!

Childcare centres will adopt an integrated curriculum framework and introduce a teacher-child ratio to ensure sufficient trained teachers.

The Government will provide recurrent grants for eligible not-for-profit childcare centre operators to set the benchmark for quality and affordability.

From 1 Jan 2009, subsidies for centre-based childcare and infant care will increase from $150 and $400 to a maximum of $300 and a maximum of $600 per month per child respectively. This applies to all Singaporean children.

ENHANCED QUALITY OF KINDERGARTEN EDUCATION

The recurrent grant will be enhanced for eligible kindergarten operators to further improve the quality of kindergarten education. Scholarships will be awarded to deserving pre-school teachers in kindergartens.

Figure 2.2 Continued

82–83) interviewed eight Singaporean–Chinese female graduates between the ages of 27 and 38, as well as their mothers—ranging in age from 49 to 70—and found that "none of our graduate interviewees thought the financial payouts had been a decisive influence in their fertility choices." Yap (2009: 167) statistically decomposed the change in TFR over the 2000–2005 period and concluded that "the decline in marital fertility rates suggest[s] that married Singaporeans have not responded to the Government's efforts but . . . the early years of the new millennium were an especially difficult period, marked by uncertainty and restructuring of the economy." These studies indicated the ineffectiveness of pronatalist incentives in encouraging childbearing behavior. However, what might explain such ineffectiveness? In general, what might be the specific linkage between macro-level state policies and micro-level individual childbearing behavior? These are empirical questions that cannot be addressed if the analysis remains at the macro level.

Perhaps more importantly, the notion of "a differential class-specific pronatalism" no longer seems relevant. Indeed, studies of Singapore's population policies tend to treat Wee's (1995) concerns as a "phase" of the past, discarded due to voters' protests and dissatisfaction. Have policy changes—regardless of intentions of policy makers—invalidated the observations by Drakakis-Smith and Graham (1996), Palen (1986) and Wee (1995) in the 1990s? How do citizens—in an environment in which citizenship entails duties and responsibilities rather than rights and entitlements—perceive and respond to the "call of duty" to reproduce (Tan and Asmani 2004)? Chapter 4 attempts to answer these questions, particularly in relation to the policies' financial incentives component.

Female labor force participation, fertility, and pronatalist policies

Cheung (1989) suggested that the increased labor force participation rate of married women helped to counter the effectiveness of pronatalist measures, and that the policies placed a high dual demand—to reproduce and to participate in the labor force—on women. Cheung further predicted that the success of new pronatalist population policies will depend largely on the willingness of women to reconcile their careers with larger family size. More recent work, however, suggested that it is important to examine how both men and women relate to pronatalist policies. For example, Jones *et al.* (2009: 187) made the following observation:

> Perhaps the most significant change in the post-2000 population policies is the ideological change regarding men's role in the family. In 2000, paternity leave [three days for fathers in the civil service] was introduced as part of the new population policies . . . [F]or the first time, men were considered to be directly involved in child care. In addition, men are now eligible to take unrecorded child care leave, which was previously only available to their female counterparts in the civil service.

Indeed, the combination of high female labor force participation and high levels of fertility has been noted in Sweden, and scholars have attributed this to the role of public policy. The empirical existence of such a successful combination suggests that it is not female labor force participation or the state's expectation of women to play a dual role as both workers and parents *per se* that explains the ineffectiveness of pronatalist policies. Given the literature on the emerging heterogeneity of life aspirations, women might aspire to be both workers and parents, as do men. They may also aspire to focus on one sphere. The kind of aspirations individuals in a group or a society have is an empirical question that needs to be investigated rather than assumed. Moreover, the Swedish case suggests the importance of public policy, but the kind of public policy that would be effective is, again, an empirical question in relation to a specific group or society. In other words, existing studies have yet to answer, for example, what, in Singapore, are women's and men's aspirations in relation to work and family life? How do career-oriented working men and women respond to the latest pronatalist policy measures supporting work-life balance? Are their responses similar to or different from the responses of family-oriented working men and women or stay-at-home parents? What can be done to allow workers to have as many children as they want? Chapter 5 attempts to answer questions raised in this section.

This study: methodological considerations

The idea behind this study's multi-stage qualitative research design is that people tell different stories about their motives and planned actions in different contexts, particularly in the contested social arenas of action and decision-making about life-altering events. Childbearing is one such decision in which peer pressure, parental intervention, and individual desire are intricately intertwined, and the role of state policy to tip the balance can best be understood by discerning connections, interactions, and feedback loops among this complex set of factors. These questions about the intersections between macro- and micro-level factors cannot be answered with de-contextualized instruments such as survey questionnaires because these survey measures are administered in an unknown and unknowable social vacuum in which feedback is necessarily and understandably assumed rather than explored and examined.

Indeed, as Ritchie and Spencer (2002: 305) explained, "the wider use of qualitative methods [in the last two decades] . . . is underpinned by the persistent requirement in social policy fields to understand complex behaviors, needs, systems, and cultures." Snowball sampling facilitated access to respondents through existing networks with built-in trust, and was considered an appropriate sampling strategy, given that previous research found that Singaporeans treat childbearing as a "private" and "personal" decision (Graham 1995; Teo and Yeoh 1999). I trained 11 research assistants who were senior university students (seven Singaporean–Chinese, two Singaporean–Indians, and two Singaporean–Malays) in interviewing techniques. Each research assistant then contacted 15 interviewees who were women of childbearing age, the target group for pronatalist population policies. For the first stage, these research assistants conducted semi-structured interviews with 165 women. Among the interviewees, 51 were married and 114 were unmarried (mostly in the 19–24 age group), as the larger project also explored the younger generation's knowledge and attitudes toward state pronatalist policies. Interviews were conducted in English, Malay, or Tamil, depending on respondents' comfort level. The length of the semistructured interviews in the first stage of the project was usually 30–45 minutes. Each interview was recorded on tape and transcribed verbatim (and translated when necessary).

Of the 165 respondents, 32 self-identified as Malays, 24 as Indians, 105 as Chinese, and 4 as "others"; 105 had received university education or were receiving such education during the interview period, and 60 did not have any university education (one interviewee did not disclose her educational level); 131 lived in government-subsidized apartments (Housing and Development Board units), and 32 lived in private properties including condominiums and landed properties (two interviewees declined to disclose their housing type). With regard to monthly household income, 40 lived in lower-income households with monthly income below S$3,000; 85 lived in middle-income households with monthly income of S$3,000–7,999; and 38 lived in higher income households with monthly income above S$8,000 (two interviewees declined to reveal their income level).

In terms of national-level data, in 2010, 23 percent of the resident non-student population aged 15 years and over had university qualifications (Singapore Department of Statistics 2011a); in 2007, 27.2 percent of employed resident households earned a monthly income of at least S$8,000; and, in 2008, 16.5 percent of employed resident households lived in private condominiums and private houses (Singapore Department of Statistics 2009a). In comparison with the national data, the average level of education of the respondents in this study is clearly higher, reflecting the participation of young, unmarried university students. Participants' dwelling types and monthly household income, however, are only slightly higher than the national distribution.

Women in the first stage nominated individuals who had or would have a significant influence on their own childbearing decision making, and these individuals were invited to participate in focus group discussions. As Morgan (1997: 46) explained:

> Until they interact with others on a topic, individuals are often simply unaware of their own implicit perspectives. Moreover, the interaction in the group may present the need to explain or defend one's perspective to someone who thinks about the world differently. Using focus groups to create such interactions gives the researcher a set of observations that is difficult to obtain through other methods.

Individuals included in the second stage were mostly husbands or boyfriends, and, in a few cases, friends of the same sex. In the third stage, focus group interviews were conducted with individual women (and/or their significant others) and their parents or parents-in-law. All participation was voluntary, and participants who joined the study in the second and third stages provided their written demographic information after the discussion. A total of 39 focus group interviews were conducted. Typically there were four to six participants in each focus group interview. Length of discussions was usually 60–90 minutes.

Sussman, Burton, Dent, and Stacy (1991) found that focus group data tended to make subjects' responses more extreme than responses offered in response to survey questionnaires. This also happened during the collection of data for this study—particularly when respondents were asked why they wanted more than one child. During face-to-face interviews, women tended to give minimal, even cryptic explanations of why they desired a specific number of children, but, then, in focus group discussions, their explanations became more elaborate and substantial as a result of questioning from other group participants.

In essence, the research design tries to approximate decision-making processes by providing appropriate settings. For the first-stage, semistructured interviews, conducted between October and December 2007, the interview schedule was divided into four sections. The first focused on the value of children. The second inquired about an individual's attitudes and opinions about marriage and paid employment. The third elicited responses to the government's pronatalist policies and the fourth collected respondents' demographic information (see Appendix B). With regard to focus group interviews in the second and third stages, conducted from January to July 2008, discussion revolved around four central questions:

1. The role of the baby bonus (or childcare subsidy) in the decision to have an additional child.
2. The role of education subsidies in decisions to have a(nother) child.
3. The degree to which availability of public housing influenced the decision-making process.
4. The ideal balance between work and family life for a couple.

Including all three stages, 204 interviews were carried out from October 2007 to July 2008, involving 221 Singaporean interviewees. Of these, 36 were men and 185 women. The average age of respondents was 29 years. A total of 84 respondents were married, and 137 were unmarried; 42 self-identified as Malays, 42 as Indians, 133 as Chinese, and 4 as "others"; 128 respondents had received or were receiving university education during the interview period, and 93 did not have any university education; 176 respondents lived in government-subsidized apartments (Housing and Development Board units), and 43 lived in private properties including private condominiums/flats and landed properties (two interviewees declined to disclose their housing type). Finally, in terms of monthly household income, 52 lived in lower-income households with monthly income below S$3,000; 112 lived in middle-income households with monthly income of S$3,000–7,999; and 53 lived in higher-income households with monthly income above S$8,000 (two interviewees declined to reveal their income level).

Data analysis

All 204 interviews were audiotaped, transcribed, and translated. As Berg (2009: 148) wrote regarding the analysis of data obtained from interviews:

> typically, a systematic indexing process begins as researchers set up several sheets of paper with major topics of interest listed separately. . . . Ideally, this process should be accomplished by two or more researchers/coders, independently reading and coding each of several transcripts.

In addition to coding all background variables and answers to close-ended survey questions, all content from the 204 interviews was coded independently by three coding teams (including five research assistants and the author) according to the following criteria, with specific page numbers in the transcripts and exact phrasing:

1. Whether and how respondents mentioned costs of living as a concern (binary coding).
2. Whether and how respondents asked for more housing subsidies.
3. Whether and how respondents asked for more educational subsidies.
4. Whether and how respondents asked for more health subsidies.
5. Whether and how respondents provide an answer to the "capstone" question: has the government made it easier financially for people to have children? Answers are coded as a) positive, b) mixed (e.g., "to some extent"), and c) negative.
6. Respondents' level of knowledge of pronatalist policies regarding financial incentives, work–life balance, and other policies: a) details (e.g., amount of the financial incentives or month entitled for maternity leave), b) keywords, and c) unaware.
7. Respondents' feedback regarding cash benefits, tax rebates, and the Children's Development Account: a) positive, b) reserved/mixed, c) negative, and d) unaware.
8. Whether and how respondents mentioned job insecurity (in general) as a concern.
9. Whether and how respondents mentioned job insecurity (in relation to family leave-taking) as a concern.
10. Respondents' feedback towards existing maternity leave: a) positive, b) negative, and c) no comment.
11. Respondents' feedback toward existing paternity leave: a) positive, b) negative, and c) no comment.
12. Whether and how respondents expressed a desire for flexible work hours.
13. Whether and how respondents expressed a desire for onsite childcare.
14. Whether and how respondents expressed a desire for homemaker allowances.
15. Whether and how respondents mention that they want their children to "be the best" or that they would "give the best" to their children to enhance their competitive edge.
16. Whether and how respondents describe their desire to provide their children with a sibling.

We then met to discuss our coding so that the whole data set could be recorded into one master index sheet and entered into the quantitative and qualitative analysis computer software. Where there were disagreements over which category to assign for any given respondent, the decision was to:

1. follow the majority (when one coder disagreed with the other two coders); or
2. to reach a consensus after discussion (when each coder assigned a different code).

Most responses were recorded straightforwardly into the master copy and the computer software programs because codes assigned were identical among the coders. I examined patterns in the data from the 165 women and analyzed themes of the focus group interviews to flesh out and explore possible explanations for patterns observed in the 165 interviews. As Bailey (2007: 153, 159) explained, "themes are recurring patterns, topics, viewpoints, emotions, concepts, events, and so on," and "a thematic analysis is at its strongest when the themes are conceptual categories and relationships among themes are explored."

In the following chapters, participants are referred to by pseudonyms for reasons of confidentiality. Married respondents are given the honorifics "Mr." and "Mrs.," while unmarried respondents are referred to by first names. When quoting from the data, I retain the original words of the respondents, including words in "Singlish"—a local version of English—and provide clarification where necessary. Before we delve into the findings, however, it is necessary to understand the development of Singapore.

3 Economic development, social investments, and population control

> Victorian England and Stalinist Russia did not present pretty pictures of bucolic happiness when they went through the process of capital accumulation and there is no reason to expect that the backward countries of the world can hope to escape the same traumatic experience if they want to achieve self-sustaining economic growth . . . To me, this rather than the technical problems of economic planning, is the real dilemma facing Asian countries today . . . The integrated, comprehensive, all embracing approach to these vital problems of the modernization process has yet to be made.
>
> Goh Keng Swee 1972, *The Economics of Modernization*

Singapore: "from Third World to first"

Singapore's economic success has been phenomenal. In less than half a century, the nation-state has transformed from a place plagued by the "unemployed or underemployed, undernourished, and inadequately housed"[1] to a "healthy, educated, and wealthy nation" (Low and Aw 1997). This success story has garnered international attention and drawn scholarly examination. As economic development is deemed to be of central importance in understanding Singapore, the first part of this chapter uses macro-level economic indicators to review its signature achievement, and draws on existing work that highlights the export-led, foreign-capital-intensive character of its development. More importantly, however, this chapter is concerned with a set of domestic institutions and state practices integral to Singapore's economic development—specifically, the leadership of the People's Action Party (PAP), with its emphasis on state expenditure on education to cultivate human resources while controlling expenditure in other areas (such as social security, housing, and health) through institutional mechanisms, most notably the Central Provident Fund (CPF) and Housing Development Board (HDB). These "developmental" and "productivist" mechanisms, I suggest, discourage economically unproductive behaviour by emphasizing that welfare is primarily the citizen's responsibility, not the state's; the state assists those who are proven least able to help themselves. Furthermore, this chapter suggests that state population policies—from anti-natalist to pronatalist—also form a fundamental part of the government's "all embracing approach" to the pursuit of economic development.

To begin, Singapore's success is best captured by the title of a book by Lee Kuan Yew, the first prime minister of the nation—*From Third World to First: The Singapore Story: 1965–2000*. Singapore's dramatic transformation from independence in 1965 to the present can be seen through a series of macro-level economic indicators. For example, as shown in Table 3.1, its real GDP has increased 100-fold since independence—from approximately S$3 billion (US$964 million) in 1965 to S$304 billion (US$223 billion) in 2010; its per-capita GDP has increased 34-fold during the same period—from approximately S$1,580 (US$516) in 1965 to S$59,813 (US$43,867) in 2010. Singapore's foreign reserve has also grown consistently—at S$289 billion in 2010 it is 236 times the 1965 amount (approximately S$12 million). Foreign equity investment in Singapore has also grown, from S$13 billion in 1980 to approximately S$464 billion in 2008. The GDP growth rate from 1960 to 2008 averaged 7 percent (Singapore Department of Statistics, *Yearbook of Statistics* various years).

Most remarkably, such achievements have been accomplished with low unemployment rates; the rates have been generally below 5 percent (Bercuson 1995). As noted in Chapter 1, government social expenditures on education, health, medical, and housing as a percentage of GDP have also generally been kept relatively low. The government's financial situation changed from a deficit of S$80 million in 1965 to a surplus of S$15.4 billion in 2010 (Singapore Department of Statistics various years, *Yearbook of Statistics*).

Export-led and foreign-capital-intensive economic development

Blomqvist (2005) summed up the history of Singapore as such:

> When Singapore was ousted from the Federation of Malaysia in 1965, it lost its natural hinterland, the Malay Peninsula. Moreover, during the last years of the Soekarno era, Indonesia had launched its policy of "confrontation," which was detrimental to the entrepot activities based in Singapore. Finally, Britain announced the impending dismantling of its military bases in Singapore . . . Any inward-looking strategy was out of the question after Singapore left the Malaysian federation . . . Industrialization took off only after independence and as a result of deliberate policy with the state as the major "entrepreneur" . . . [T]he characteristic trait of Singapore's industrialization process was the country's reliance on foreign capital—multinational companies (MNCs) rather than domestic players.

Indeed, the role of foreign capital and multinational corporations in the growth of Singapore's economy cannot be overemphasized. Low (2006) described Singapore's three phases of economic development as "Singapore Incorporated" (1959–1968), "Singapore International" (1969–1992), and "Singapore Unlimited" (1993–present). The role of MNCs has been critical in each phase: in the first, it was "active state-owned enterprise on one hand and infusion of foreign direct investment and MNCs on the other"; in the second, "both MNCs and GLCs [i.e.,

Table 3.1 Key Indicators of Singapore's Economic Performance (1965–2010)

Year	*Real GDP[a] S$m (US$ mil)*	*Per capita GDP[b] S$ (US$)*	*General govt. finance[c] S$m [deficit(–) or surplus]*	*Foreign reserve[c] S$m*	*Foreign equity investment[d] S$m*	*Unemployment rate[e] (percent)*
1965	2,982.2 (974.2)	1,580 (516)	–80.3	1,224.4	N.A.	N.A.
1970	5,876 (1,919.5)	2,832 (925)	78.9	3,097.9	N.A.	6
1975	13,722.3 (5,786.8)	6,065 (2,558)	141.9	7,486	N.A.	4.6
1980	25,792.6 (12,045.9)	10,685 (4,990)	407.4	13,757.7	13,002.4	3.5
1985	40,622.1 (18,462.9)	14,847 (6,748)	N.A.	27,080.1	25,502.7	4.2
1990	70,390.6 (38,836.2)	23,101 (12,745)	6225.7	48,521.3	57,935.2	1.3
1995	123,399.8 (87,060.7)	35,012 (24,702)	14825.9	97,336.6	99,215.7	2
2000	162,584.1 (94,311.8)	40,364 (23,414)	13657.9	139,260	189,118	2.7
2005	208,763.7 (125,413.7)	48,939 (29,400)	13397.5	192,813	316,651	3.1

Continued

Table 3.1 Continued

Year	*Real GDP[a] S$m (US$ mil)*	*Per capita GDP[b] S$ (US$)*	*General govt. finance[c] S$m [deficit(–) or surplus]*	*Foreign reserve[c] S$m*	*Foreign equity investment[d] S$m*	*Unemployment rate[e] (percent)*
2006	230,922.8 (145,335)	52,466 (33,020)	21017.7	208,991.8	372,368	2.7
2007	267,253.5 (177,329.6)	58,243 (38,646)	29768.3	234,545.6	461,727	2.1
2008	267,951.9 (189,392.1)	55,369 (39,136)	24100.1	250,346	464,347	2.2
2009	266,659.2 (183,333.9)	53,464 (36,758)	–4,357.6[4]	263,955.4	N.A.	3.0
2010	303,652.2 (222,700.6)	59,813 (43,867)	15433.6[4]	288,954.1[f]	N.A.	2.2

Sources:

a Singapore Department of Statistics (2011c)
b Singapore Department of Statistics (2011d)
c Singapore Department of Statistics, *Yearbook of Statistics*
d Adapted from Singapore Department of Statistics (2010b)
e Adapted from Ministry of Manpower (2011b)
f Adapted from Monetary Authority of Singapore (2011)

Government Linked Companies] [were] spearheaded further outside the domestic company"; and the current phase is represented by "Singapore's desire to induce MNCs outside the region wishing to tap Asia Pacific, to use Singapore as the base and conduit." As of 2007, there were 7,000 MNCs and 100,000 small and medium enterprises (SMEs) in Singapore; of these companies, more than 4,000 have established their headquarters in Singapore (Economic Development Board 2007).

As shown in Tables 3.2 and 3.3, the importance of the manufacturing industry increased continuously during the years 1965–1990, but has declined since then, signaling Singapore's transition to a post-industrial society. Concomitantly, the service sector—particularly communication, financial, and business services—has gained increasing prominence in terms of both contribution to the GDP and share of the labor market.

As Singapore's economic performance has been exceptionally brilliant, what are some of the key domestic institutions and institutional mechanisms that have contributed to such success?

The People's Action Party

The People's Action Party (PAP), formed in late 1954, was first elected to the ruling position of governance in 1959. Elections were competitive in the 1950s and 1960s, but, by 1968, the PAP had survived serious political competition and emerged as a hegemonic party, winning every parliamentary seat until 1981, when a by-election broke the monopoly (Chua 1995). However, the PAP's ruling position has not been threatened, as the opposition—such as The Worker's Party, National Solidarity Party, Singapore People's Party, and Singapore Democratic Alliance—has managed to win only two or three seats, at most, until the General Election in 2011, in which the opposition gained six seats.[2] George (2010: 261) explained PAP's dominance this way:

> It is helpful to think of Singapore as a networked autocracy . . . Authoritarian regimes are conventionally associated with a high risk of calamitous collapse, because they tend to become increasingly unresponsive to citizens' needs and preferences. It is the networked quality of Singapore's authoritarian model that may account for its exceptional resilience. Unlike most highly centralized states, Singapore's regime has kept itself open and connected—to its mass base to which it remains highly responsive, to elites whom it works hard to co-opt, and to global economic forces with which its policies are kept in tune. Such openness does not amount to democracy as widely understood, since the PAP has erected formidable barriers to political competition. However, the government has instituted increasingly elaborate systems to ensure its responsiveness to the nation's needs. The internet has been harnessed as part of that system, with agencies creating their own online feedback channels, as well as monitoring discussions in the rest of cyberspace.

Indeed, the PAP government's legitimacy is primarily derived from its success in fostering continuous economic growth and improving the general material lives

Table 3.2 Industry output as a percentage of GDP (1965–2009)

Sector	*1965*	*1970*	*1975*	*1980*	*1985*	*1990*
	Percent					
Total	100	100	100	100	100	100
Manufacturing	15.1	20.4	24.1	29.5	24.6	29.5
Construction	6.3	6.8	8.1	6.7	11.0	5.7
Utilities[a]	2.2	2.6	1.9	2.4	2.1	2.0
Other goods industries[b]	3.2	2.7	2.3	1.7	1.1	0.4
Transport, storage, and communications	11.4	10.8	11.3	12.5	14.1	13.3
Wholesale, retail trade, restaurants, and hotels (trade) [d]	27.5	28.2	27.0	24.3	18.5	17.2
Financial and business services[c]	8.8	9.0	14.6	16.3	23.1	28.0
Others	25.4	19.4	10.7	6.6	5.5	3.9

Sector	*1995*	*2000*	*2005*	*2006*	*2007*	*2008*	*2009*
	Percent						
Total	100	100	100	100	100	100	100
Manufacturing	26.3	26.5	25.4	25.6	23.3	19.5	18.5
Construction	7.1	6.1	3.6	3.4	3.7	5.1	5.1
Utilities[a]	1.6	1.7	1.7	1.7	1.6	1.4	1.3
Other goods industries[b]	0.2	0.1	0.1	0.1	0.1	0.1	0.04
Transport, storage, and communications	11.6	11.3	13.8	13	12.7	12.8	12.1
Wholesale, retail trade, restaurants, and hotels (trade) [d]	19.4	19.6	18.7	19.8	19.2	19.3	18.8
Financial and business services[c]	29.6	25.9	22.2	22.6	24.5	27.2	24.9
Others	4.2	8.8	14.5	13.9	15	14.4	19.26

Source: Singapore Department of Statistics, *Yearbook of Statistics*, various years.

Notes

a Labeled as "Electricity, gas and water" in sources for years 1965 and 1970.

b Labeled as "Agriculture and fishing" and "quarrying" in sources for years 1965–1980.

c Labeled as "Finance, insurance, real estate, and business services" in sources for years 1965 and 1970.

d Labeled as "Trade" in sources for years 1975–1980, "Commerce" for years 1985–1995.

of its citizens (Chua 1995). It has been able to deliver economic progress effectively through the expansion of state institutions (e.g., the Government of Singapore Investment Corporation, the Elected President Scheme, the Nominated Member of Parliament Scheme, the Group Representation Constituencies, etc.), thereby enhancing its legitimacy to rule (Ho 2010). Moreover, as early as the 1960s, the government saw an imperative to modernize through attracting multinational

Table 3.3 Industry share of the labor market (1969–2009)

	1969	*1970*	*1975*	*1980*	*1985*	*1990*	*1995*	*2000*	*2005*	*2006*	*2007*	*2008*	*2009*
	Percent												
Total	100	100	100	100	100	100	100	100	100	100	100	100	100
Manufacturing	27.5	29.9	26.2	30.1	25.4	29.1	24.2	19.5	16.7	16.8	16.9	16.8	15.7
Construction	5.3	5.0	4.7	6.7	8.9	7.9	6.7	6.1	5	5.3	5.6	5.7	6.1
Services	62.9	61.1	65.3	60.7	63.9	62.1	67.8	73.5	77.3	76.7	76.4	76.2	77.1
Commerce[a]	22.4	22.5	23.0	21.3	23.5	22.0	20.4	23.4	18.4	23.9	22.2	21	21.3
Transport, storage, information, and communication	9.6	9.5	11.7	11.1	10.1	9.5	10.7	13.9	13.8	13.8	14.8	14.5	14.7
Financial and business services	30.9	5.5	6.1	7.4	8.7	10.9	14.6	17.2	18.8	18	18.5	19.5	19.5
Community, social, and personal services		23.6	24.5	20.9	21.5	19.7	22.1	19	20	20.9	20.8	21.2	21.6
Others[b]	4.3	4.0	3.8	2.5	1.8	0.8	1.2	0.9	1.1	1.3	1.1	1.2	1.1

Source: Singapore, Department of Statistics, *Yearbook of Statistics*, various years.

Notes

a “Commerce” includes wholesale, retail trade, hotels, and restaurants.

b “Others” include agriculture, fishing, quarrying, utilities, and activities not adequately defined.

corporations (MNCs), which, at the time, were searching for new, low-cost manufacturing centers. The strategy has been to create a conducive investment climate for foreign investment. According to Tremewan (1998: 81), Singapore's attractiveness to foreign capital was a package, which included:

> A continuing supply of relatively cheap, disciplined workers with appropriate skills, a relatively developed infrastructure being rapidly improved, a state policy constantly to upgrade the technical level of production, a strategic geographical location, and a reliable government administration whose governance was largely uncontested by the end of 1960s.

Similarly, Chew (1994: 939–940) suggested that two conditions have been crucial for foreign investment in Singapore: political stability and a low wage, non-militant workforce. How has the PAP-led government successfully created a low-wage and highly-disciplined labor force? It has done so through a series of legislative and political measures; for instance, it has effectively controlled the workforce by making changes in labor laws and labor-related institutions, at the same time, it has enhanced social discipline of the workforce through provisions of public welfare.

Changes in labor laws have restricted union activity. For instance, in August 1966, "the Trade Union (Amendment) Bill made it illegal for any union to strike or take other industrial actions without the consent of the majority of its members" (Chua 1995: 18). The Industrial Relations (Amendment) Act (1968) further restricted union activity, removing rights to address issues of hiring, firing, promotions, and work assignments. Union activity was eventually taken up by the National Trade Union Congress (NTUC), a newly created national-level labor union that enjoyed the patronage of the government and adhered to government policies (Chew 1994).

To control wage levels, the task of wage bargaining has been delegated to the National Wage Council (NWC)—an institution representing employers, the NTUC, and the government—which sets national guidelines for wage adjustment each year. As Tremewan noted (Tremewan 1998: 82):

> although the NWC has been referred to as a tripartite body, with the Secretary-General of the NTUC being a member of the cabinet, it has been, in effect, a coordinating body of the PAP-government and foreign capital to regulate the core of their partnership.

The NWC has played a significant role in adjusting wage levels according to the government's economic strategies, notably to suppress wage levels in the late 1960s to attract foreign investment, and then to ensure orderly wage increases in the 1980s, in line with the PAP's strategy to upgrade the economy (Chua 1999). The PAP government's success in regulating wages and disciplining the labor force was also achieved through its provision of public goods and services, which will be elaborated upon in the next section.

Institutionalizing citizen-responsibility through compulsory savings

Singapore's economic development strategy is critically linked to its domestic institutions—in particular, the Central Provident Fund (CPF), which embodies the notion of citizenship-as-responsibility. The CPF, established by the colonial administration in 1953, became operative in 1955 as a straightforward savings and withdrawal retirement plan; 5 percent of an employee's wage was compulsorily saved, and an equivalent amount contributed by the employer. The fund has evolved and the CPF board now explains it in the following way (CPF, 1995: 19):

> Each month, both employer and employee contribute to the employee's CPF savings which earn interest . . . The contributions are tax free. The rate of contribution is 40 percent of the salary—20 percent from the member, and 20 percent from the employer. The amount from each is capped at $1,200 based on a monthly salary of $6,000.

Compulsory rates of contribution have changed substantially over the years, according to the government's economic developmental goals. For instance, when Singapore had its first severe recession and its real GDP declined by 1.6 percent in 1985, the government managed to maintain its long-term goal of economic growth by reducing employers' contribution to the CPF from 25 to 10 percent. Moreover, since 1955, "it [the CPF] has evolved from a simple compulsory [retirement] savings scheme into a comprehensive social security savings plan providing for the retirement, healthcare, and housing needs of Singaporeans" (CPF 2005: 9). Indeed, the CPF has gradually become multipurpose: members have been able to use their CPF savings to pay for public housing since 1968 (e.g. the Public Housing Scheme), to pay for their dependents' as well as their own hospitalization expenses from 1984 (e.g. the Medisave Scheme), and to finance tertiary education in Singapore for themselves or their children from 1989 (e.g. the Education Scheme). In January 1987, the government instituted the "Minimum Sum Scheme" for CPF contribution; each member is required to set aside a certain amount in their CPF account. The idea was that such a Minimum Sum would give members "a regular income after the official retirement age." This sum was set at S$80,000 in 2003, to be raised to S$120,000 (in 2003 dollars) in 2013.

While the CPF's reach has been extended, one principle has not changed: "the CPF is entirely funded by the workers themselves and their employers" (Ramesh 2004: 63; see also Holliday 2003: 73). CPF ratios of contribution are shown in Table 3.4 and Table 3.5, and its key schemes are shown in Appendix C.

Citizens, as CPF account holders, earn interest on their CPF balances, while investment of CPF balances "is the primary responsibility of the Government of Singapore Investment Corporation (GIC), which is a private limited company wholly owned by the Singapore government . . . This in effect lends members savings to the government" (Asher and Newman 2001). Similarly, Tremewan (1998: 85) noted:

Table 3.4 Combined employer/employee contribution rates to the Singapore Central Provident Fund by age and plan account (percent)

Age (from)	*Long term target*				*2011*			
	Ordinary	*Special*	*Medisave*	*Total*	*Ordinary*	*Special*	*Medisave*	*Total*
22.0	30.0	4.0	6.0	40.0	23.0	5.5	7.0	35.5
35.0	29.0	4.0	7.0	40.0	21.0	6.5	8.0	35.5
45.0	28.0	4.0	8.0	40.0	19.0	7.5	9.0	35.5
55.0	12.0	0.0	8.0	20.0	11.5	0.5	9.0	21.0
60.0	7.0	0.0	8.0	15.0	3.5	0.5	9.5	13.5
65.0	2.0	0.0	8.0	10.0	1.0	0.5	9.5	11.0

Source:
McCarthy *et al.* (2002)

> Since then [1986] the [CPF] interest rate has been calculated as the average rate of that offered by four major local banks, still a comparatively low figure (3.1 percent in 1995) . . . Therefore, during the process of industrialization, the Singapore government has had access to a huge flow of cheap capital for infrastructural development including public housing and has not needed to raise foreign loans. The CPF had 417,000 contributors in 1966 with total compulsory savings of more than S$400 million . . . The end of 1995 saw the total savings swell to S$66 billion with 2.69 million CPF members.

CPF contributions stood at approximately S$182 billion (or precisely S$181,712.1 million) with 3.33 million CPF members as of September 2010 (CPF 2011). More recently, in the context of international pressure for liberalization and deregulation, Rodan (2004: 53) commented that:

> up to a point, the [Singapore] government has been responsive here, parcelling out portions of the CPF to private fund managers. However, it is reluctant to surrender fundamental control over the CPF because through it a range of social policies are enacted. Indeed, *the government increasingly deploys the CPF to foster self-funded health, educational and social security investments* (my emphasis).

In summary, the CPF is simultaneously a mechanism to ensure welfare provisions, which are tied to individual citizens' paid employment, and a macroeconomic tool for the state.

The government has also been able to keep a lid on citizens' usage of various self-financed CPF accounts through administrative rules and regulations. For example, regulation of usage of citizens' accounts for healthcare expenses is carried out primarily through three mechanisms: the "Medisave Minimum Sum" scheme, "the Medisave Required Amount" scheme, and rules limiting withdrawal to cover hospital

Table 3.5 CPF contribution rates (1955–2011)

Year	*Contribution by employee*	*Contribution by employer*	*Total*
1955	5.0	5.0	10.0
1968	6.5	6.5	13.0
1970	8.0	8.0	16.0
1971	10.0	10.0	20.0
1972	10.0	14.0	24.0
1973	11.0	15.0	26.0
1974	15.0	15.0	30.0
1977	15.5	15.5	31.0
1978	16.5	16.5	33.0
1979	16.5	20.5	37.0
1980	18.0	20.5	38.5
1981	22.0	20.5	42.5
1982	23.0	22.0	45.0
1983	23.0	23.0	46.0
1984	25.0	25.0	50.0
1986	25.0	10.0	35.0
1988	24.0	12.0	36.0
1989	23.0	15.0	38.0
1990	23.0	16.5	39.5
1991	22.5	17.5	40.0
1992	22.0	18.0	40.0
1994	20.0	20.0	40.0
1999	20.0	10.0	30.0
2000	20.0	12.0	32.0
2001	20.0	16.0	36.0
2002	20.0	16.0	36.0
2003	20.0	13.0	33.0
2004	20.0	13.0	33.0
2005	20.0	13.0	33.0
2006	20.0	13.0	33.0
2007	20.0	14.5	34.5
2011	20.0	15.5	35.5

Sources:
Central Provident Fund (2005b) and Tremewan (1998)

bills. The withdrawal limit rules, in particular, have direct implications for how much parents and prospective parents have to pay for medical expenses out of their own pockets rather than through the CPF Medisave account. For instance, withdrawal limits stipulate that "for a hospitalization claim, the patient must have stayed in the hospital for at least 8 hours (unless the patient is admitted for day surgery) or died within 8 hours of being hospitalized," and that "Medisave covers up to $450 per day for daily hospital charges . . . a fixed limit per table of surgical operations." In other words, while citizens can draw on their Medisave account to make payments, there will almost always be a proportion to be paid in cash.

In addition, there is a complex system of state health service provision, including a five-tier series of ward subsidies,[3] a ratio of ward classes within hospitals, and an overall revenue cap on the amount hospitals can charge patients per episode of treatment. The result of this complex system, according to Holliday, is that

> government health expenditure amounted to about 26 percent of total health-care spending in 2000. The rest of the spending was contributed by individuals through Medisave accounts and out-of-pocket expenses, and by insurance companies inside or outside the Medisave system.
>
> (2003: 90–91; see also Ramesh 2004: 108)

With regard to usage of CPF accounts for educational purposes, the government explains:

> The CPF Education Scheme is a loan scheme. The total amount withdrawn for tuition fees plus accrued interest has to be repaid in full with cash. Repayment will start one year after date of graduation or date of leaving the institution, whichever is earlier. Interest starts accruing from the day of withdrawal, and is pegged to the prevailing CPF Ordinary Account interest rate which is currently 2.5% p.a.
>
> (CPF 2008, emphasis in original)

While the CPF is a self-funded personal account for employed citizens, this is not to suggest that there is no state-provided benefit at all. Indeed, Finance Minister Tharman Shanmugaratnam announced a 6.6 billion "wealth-sharing" budget on February 18, 2011, which was reported to be "the most generous in years," including:

> S$3.2 billion in cash gifts, bonuses and rebates to be paid out to individuals and families . . . S$1.5 billion in Growth Dividends for 2.5 million citizens, $580 million in personal income tax rebates, $224 million in Workfare Special Bonus payouts to 400,000 older, low-wage workers, and more than $100 million in Child Development Credits and subsidies for families with young children. All the payouts are tiered so that those with lower incomes receive more.
>
> (Lim, *Straits Times* February 19, 2011)

In fact, as Ramesh (2004: 54) pointed out:

> since the mid-1990s, the government has periodically 'topped up' Medisave Accounts and offered 'one-off' across the board tax allowances. A rebate of 10 percent on individual income tax was offered in 1997, 5 percent in 1998, and 10 percent in 1999. In 2000, the government topped up all CPF accounts by between S$500 and S$1,700, with the highest amount for low-income earners.

More recently, the state started to channel funding through community organizations. As Chua (2007: 36) noted, "in the 2005 annual national budget, a Community Care (Comcare) Endowment fund of S$500 million is allocated for social welfare expenditures; this is likely to generate more than $50 million a year for expenditure." The key to understanding such state action, however, as Ramesh (2004: 54) suggested, is that "they are discretionary payments that do not impose long-term commitment on the government."

Certainly, this emphasis on individual responsibility can be seen not only through the financing structure of the CPF, but also official rhetoric on various aspects of social provisions. Out of numerous examples of such rhetoric, below are a few that are directly related to social provisions. Minister Mentor Lee Kuan Yew commented on the origin of CPF in the following way:

> A universal problem we had to resolve was retirement benefits or pensions when a worker became too old to work. In Europe and America, the government provided these pensions, paid for by taxpayers. We decided that every worker should accumulate his own savings in the CPF for old age.
>
> (CPF 2005b, p. 7)

In his message on the CPF 50th anniversary website, the Minister for Manpower Dr. Ng Eng Hen said, "At the heart of it, the CPF is an institution that promotes self-reliance for individuals and their families."

A white paper issued by the Ministry for Health in 1993 explained:

> we owe it to ourselves individually to keep fit and healthy. The healthcare system needs to be structured to strengthen this sense of personal responsibility. It must give the individual maximum incentive to stay healthy, save for his medical expense and avoid using more medical services then he absolutely needs.
>
> (Ministry of Health 1993: 2)

While the Singapore government's expenditures on education and health declined from 4.5 percent of GDP in 1970 to 3.7 percent of GDP in 2008, resident household expenditures on these services have increased over the years—for instance, during 1988–2003, expenditures on housing increased from 17.5 percent to 22.4 percent, on education from 4.7 percent to 7.8 percent, and, finally, on healthcare from 2.6 percent to 5.1 percent (Singapore Department of Statistics 2003).

CPF and HDB: expending "homeownership"

The CPF scheme and the Housing Development Board (HDB) have further contributed to the creation of a low cost and highly disciplined workforce in Singapore. Formed in 1960, the HDB functions to provide public housing flats at low cost. In 1964 the HDB introduced the Home Ownership Scheme to encourage long-term leasing ("ownership") of public-sector dwellings. However, few citizens could afford the down-payment of approximately 20 percent of a flat's value. It was only in 1968, when CPF members were able to use CPF savings to finance down-payments and loans on HDB flats, that the proportion of tenants deciding to buy their flats started to increase, from 44 percent in 1968, to 63 percent in 1970, and 90 percent in 1986. As CPF savings could not otherwise be withdrawn until retirement, the option of purchasing a state-subsidized flat was immediately attractive (Tremewan 1998: 88).

The effect of CPF-financed low-cost public housing was multi-fold. First, as Tremewan (p. 90) explained:

> The relatively high cost of housing and its link to the forced saving regime of the CPF have compelled a high level of social discipline in that people have had to remain in formal employment in order to meet increasing costs and to provide for their future subsistence. Two or more household members may need to pool their incomes in order to meet housing costs. Thus the CPF and HDB have, in tandem, given strong momentum to the proletarianisation or the population, putting people physically in their places for the state's economic strategy and making their labour available to foreign capital.

The role of the state institutions of the CPF and HDB in the provision of social services while maintaining minimal government expenditures is best elucidated by Chua (2007):

> The CPF, an individualized compulsory monthly social security savings program, provides an effective financial mechanism or circuit that facilitates the expansion of homeownership while the HDB acts as both the vendor and mortgage lender to any household which is eligible to purchase a public housing flat. Members of the household, individually or collectively, can utilize their CPF savings to pay the monthly mortgage. The transfer of funds is conducted administratively between the CPF and the HDB. The entire process is conducted in a closed circuit of transactions—the working population save in their CPF, the government borrows from the CPF for infrastructure development including loans and grants to the HDB, the HDB sells the public housing, which is paid by the households monthly through deductions from their CPF—without involving any conventional banking and financial instruments. Once this mode of mortgage payment is instituted, immediately, the ratio of those who applied to purchase the ninety-nine-year lease went up rapidly. By the early 1990s, more than 85 percent of the resident population lived in HDB flats and an equal percentage of these "own" a ninety-nine-year lease on their flats.

Indeed, as Chua (2000: 47) pointed out:

> one of the boldest steps taken by the PAP government towards securing its political support base was to embark on a national public housing programme; improvement of housing conditions was a covenant between the newly enfranchised electorate and the elected government.

Housing provision is regulated by the HDB, and eligibility rules of application are based primarily on citizenship, age, family nucleus status, and income ceiling. For instance, an applicant must be a Singaporean citizen who is at least 21 years old at the time of application. The applicant's family nucleus must comprise at least one other Singaporean citizen or Singaporean permanent resident. To buy a three-room apartment, the individual citizen's gross monthly household income must not be more than S$3,000, and, to buy a three-room premium, four-room, or bigger HDB apartment, the applicant's gross monthly household income must not be more than S$8,000. In other words, state-subsidized HDB apartments aim to cater to lower- and middle-income Singaporean households.

In addition, the HDB sets the prices of apartments offered to first-time buyers, which follow market prices. According to Abeysinghe and Gu (2010: 11):

> Since 1980, the average annual growth of private residential property prices was about 11 per cent, with prices increasing, on a year-on-year basis, by 102 percent in 1981Q1, 47 percent in 1994Q3 and 31 percent in 2007Q4. The price of HDB resale flats has followed similar cycles.

In other words, HDB prices have risen rapidly over the years. In 2008, median resale prices for one- and two-room HDB apartments were below S$200,000, and prices for three-room to executive apartments were S$235,000–445,000. If citizens do not have sufficient cash, they can finance the purchase by using their CPF ordinary accounts or taking a loan from the HDB or the bank. If citizens take a loan from the HDB, there are HDB loan interest payments to be made. Finally, if citizens want to sell their apartment and upgrade to a bigger one, they have to pay a resale levy to the HDB. Teo (2010: 344) showed that "in the process of negotiating HDB rules, CPF regulations and ROM [Register of Marriage] requirements, people talk to friends, co-workers, families . . . There is an extraordinary degree of consensus about 'normal' ways to be [a Singaporean]."

In summary, with regard to the electorate, although the PAP's legitimacy to govern is taken less for granted, Singaporeans' dependency on the state's provision of public goods and services, particularly public housing and pensions, governed, respectively, by the bodies of the HDB and CPF, served to foster "commitment to the prevalent social order by the development of personal stakes in its survival." Thus, it is suggested that the PAP has achieved political hegemony:

> Where the state is able to determine the terms of public discussion regarding collective consumption goods provision, it may be said to have achieved political hegemony/consensus among the governed. This condition is empirically observable when public complaints are overwhelmingly of the type that attempt to make the agencies more efficient in serving the population, rather than involving issues of principle.
>
> (Chua 1995: 145)

Human resources development as the engine of economic growth

Another key state institution that has attracted close examination is Singapore's educational system. According to Kang (2005: 2), "Since the inception of nationhood in 1965, the government has been firmly committed to two dominant ideological pillars—meritocracy and multiracialism. One without another, and the economic miracle that is present-day Singapore would not exist." Indeed, Minister Mentor Lee Kuan Yew (2000: 288) articulated Singapore's success thus:

> Singapore set out to become a multiracial society of equal citizens, where opportunities are equal and a person's contribution is recognised and rewarded on merit, regardless of race, language, culture, or religion. In spite of our meagre natural resources, we succeeded, and our policies have benefited all our citizens, including our Malays. We have a growing middle class of professionals, executives, and businessmen, including Malays, who have developed a strong competitive spirit and take pride in being what they are on their own merit. Every time we are rated as the best airline in Asia, the No. 1 airport, the No. 1 container port, it reminds Singaporeans what a cohesive meritocratic multiracial society can achieve, better than if we were a Chinese-dominated one and lacked solidarity. This is not what Malaysia's leaders thought would happen when they asked us to leave in 1965.

What does "merit" mean? In theory, meritocracy is a system of individual social mobility based on achievement rather than ascribed status. Kang explained:

> the education system of Singapore is structured deliberately so as to allow students, regardless of ethnic group, gender or socioeconomic status, an equal opportunity to access quality educational resources . . . In this meritocratic context, examinations become the sole indicator of "merit".
>
> (Kang 2005: 7).

In the Singaporean school system, there are three major examinations: the Primary School Leaving Examination (PSLE), the Singapore-Cambridge General Certificate of Education Ordinary Level (GCE O-Level) examination, and the Singapore-Cambridge General Certificate of Education Advanced Level (GCE A-Level) examination. In other words, there are major national examinations at the end of the primary, secondary, and junior college years. Institutional features key to built-in competition in the education system, which generate concern and anxiety among parents and students, as discussed in Chapters 4 and 6, need to be further elaborated here to facilitate understanding: (a) streaming, (b) development of private education, and (c) expanded (but still limited) university enrollment.

"Streaming," instituted in 1979, is the state practice of separating primary school students into different categories ("streams") with varying academic and language curricula. At the end of the fourth grade, students are channeled into three streams—

EM1, EM2, and EM3—which indicate not only the level at which English and the mother tongue (Mandarin, Malay, and Tamil) are taught, but also putative academic abilities of pupils. English is the main language of instruction, including compulsory subjects such as science and mathematics. The curriculum for EM3 students is less rigorous than that for EM1 and EM2 students, and EM1 students are provided with instruction to learn their mother tongue at a more advanced level. Since 2004, EM1 and EM2 have been merged, and EM3 students can sit in on certain classes with EM1 and EM2 students. Streaming remains, however, a key mechanism that allows the state to sort and invest differently in students, and students to compete with one another as early as their primary school years for admission into "better" streams. Later, depending on students' PSLE results, they are placed in the Special course, Express course, Normal (Academic) course, or Normal (Technical) course in secondary school.

In addition to such internal differentiation, schools themselves are "graded." First, the Ministry of Education provides school ranking lists and achievement awards for secondary schools that perform well. Secondary schools are ranked in terms of the students' GCE O-Level scores and physical fitness. These lists have been published in local newspapers each year since 1992. In 2004 the ranking system was modified so that school performance is judged on a broader basis. Parents use information on school ranks, together with their children's PSLE results, to apply for secondary schools. There are "independent" and "autonomous" secondary schools in addition to government schools. "Independent schools" and "autonomous schools" have been set up since 1988 and 1994, respectively. These schools collect their own fees, and have more autonomy in curriculum and learning approach.

The Compulsory Education Act, implemented in 2003, requires all citizens who are above the age of 6 years and who have not yet attained the age of 15 years to enroll in a school that is part of the national education system. Moreover, in accordance with the developmental state principle noted in Chapter 1, primary and secondary school fees are nominal—except for autonomous and independent schools, which collect their own fees. Furthermore, the government established the CPF Edusave scheme in 1992, providing a set amount of money to be used for school-related activities for all students between the ages of 6 and 16 years. However, competition remains fierce, as there are national examinations at the end of primary and secondary school. Moreover, while primary school students are encouraged to participate in extracurricular activities, secondary school students' performance in co-curricular activities is taken into account for admission to higher learning institutions. Finally, as Table 3.6 shows, admission to university remains limited even though numbers of students admitted have increased over the years. In 2007, only approximately one in four students in the same Primary 1 cohort eventually made it to university.

Table 3.6 Key educational indicators (2003–2009)

Percentage of P1 cohort[a] *who*	*2003*	*2004*	*2005*	*2006*	*2007*	*2008*	*2009*
	Percent						
Sat for							
PSLE and passed	98.5	98.5	98.5	98.6	98.5	98	98.1
GCE 'N' or 'O' level examinations and had at least 5 'N' level passes or 3 'O' level passes	86.3	86.9	86.9	86.7	87.5	87.1	88.2
GCE 'A' level examinations and had at least 3 H2 passes (with a pass in GP or KI)[b]	25.3	24.6	24.7	25.2	24	25.5	25.3
Admitted into[c]							
Institute of technical education	22.2	22.1	21.5	22	20.7	21.2	21.4
Polytechnics[d]	39.3	40.1	41.5	41	42.2	42.9	42.9
Junior colleges/ centralised institutes	29.5	29.9	29.9	29.4	30.5	28	27.7
Universities (NUS, NTU, SMU)	22.4	23.2	23.8	23.9	23.6	24.8	25.4
Ratio of students to teaching staff							
Primary	24.9	24.3	23.5	22.6	21.9	21.4	19.6
Secondary	19.1	19	18.5	18.4	18.2	17.9	16.4

Source:
Ministry of Education (2010).

Notes
a The P1 cohorts represented in each year are different across the indicators, as different cohorts reach the target levels in each year.
b Figures for 2003–2006 are for at least 3 'A' level passes including GP.
c Students who enroll in one type of institution may later progress to another.
d Figures include full-time diploma students from LASELLE College of the Arts and Nanyang Academy of Fine Arts.

Education for economic development

The education system discussed above has not evolved in a vacuum; rather, it is intimately linked to Singapore's economic development strategy. Former Deputy Prime Minister and Minister of Finance Goh Keng Swee explained that the government invested financial resources "to improve and upgrade human resources, mainly by providing mass education and training for all Singaporeans, so that they [would be] ready to enter the industrial workforce" (cited in Pereira 2008). Tham (1989: 489) put it this way: "the [Singapore government's] central concern that has evoked [its] thinking and prompted its policies in education has been the matter of human resource management." Pereira (2008: 132) noted that "education in

Singapore was coordinated by the Council for Professional and Technical Education. The chairman of this council has always been the Minister for Trade and Industry."

In studying the relationship between the developmental state and the "developmental worker," Sung (2006) had the following insight:

> Education in a developmental state is not just for the purpose of imparting knowledge, or for the sake of learning. It is an important national project in which the workers in Singapore would have to cultivate a set of "collective values" necessary for industrialisation . . . Indeed, education and training soon became an important tool as the EDB [Economic Development Board] started to recruit MNCs [multinational corporations] from overseas.

Sung (2006: 55–73) divided Singapore's economic development and attendant education and training of workers into four stages: (1) 1965–1979: creating a workforce for a manufacturing base; (2) 1979–1991: beyond basic manufacturing—creating a skill-upgrading strategy; (3) 1991–1999: targeting a higher position along the value chain; and (4) 1999–present: tackling globalization and the knowledge-based economy. In each stage of development, there have been corresponding changes in the educational system. For example, Sung noted, "unlike Hong Kong, Singapore's new [economic development] strategy was not located in an economic policy document, but in an education reform report—the Goh Report (1979)." Streaming came about as a recommendation of the Goh Report. Sung argued, "the streaming system enabled the developmental state to maximise human resources as defined by the industrial policy" (Sung 2006: 57). In stage three, there were several education reforms, including the introduction of "a preparatory programme for all five-year-olds in order to compensate for the heavier demands made by the bilingual education . . . The reform shows that the rigor of learning and skill upgrading starts at an early age in Singapore" (ibid.: 63).

The development of higher learning institutions is similarly driven by economic needs envisioned by the state. For example, according to the Ministry of Trade and Industry (cited in Tan and Goh 2008: 152):

> The advanced technologies that were considered to have a big impact during this time [1990s onward] were information technology, biotechnology, robotics and artificial intelligence, microelectronics, laser technology and optics, and communication technology.

A larger pool of university graduates was deemed necessary to drive the economy forward into the 1990s. In 1991, Nanyang Technological Institute, together with the National Institute of Education, became Nanyang Technological University, Singapore's second full-fledged university, and, in 2000, Singapore Management University admitted its first class of business students.

In short, while education consistently accounts for a significant share of government expenditure, it is driven less by the aspirations of the people than the state's investment in human resources to increase productivity and fuel economic development.

Female education and labor force participation

Minister Mentor Lee Kuan Yew was also a strong proponent of mass female education. He made the following comment in a speech to women at the National Trade Union Congress (cited in Pereira 2008): "Societies which do not educate and use half their potential because they are women are those which will be worse off . . . [W]e cannot not educate and use the energy and ability of our women."

As indicated in Table 3.7, the official survey data show that women have become better educated since 1965: the literacy rate among females increased from 42.6 percent in 1965 to 93.3 percent in 2009, and mean years of schooling for females grew from 3.7 years in 1980 to 9.2 years in 2009. Moreover, female labor force participation increased from 24.2 percent in 1965 to 55.2 percent in 2009. Among working persons aged 15 and over, 43 percent were women in 2009. Even more dramatically, in 2009 close to half (50.6 percent) of working women aged 15 and over were professional, managerial, and technical workers (Ministery of Manpower 2010).

Minority education and labor force participation

While there are opportunities for every child to undergo at least ten years of general education, and school enrollment ratios for the age group 7–16 are more or less equally high among the major ethnic groups in Singapore—98.7 percent for Chinese, 97.1 percent for Malays, and 98.4 percent for Indians—there are differences in educational outcomes among these groups at the higher end of the system. For example, according to census data, among the non-student population aged 15 years and over, the Chinese have attained the most education, followed by Indians and then Malays. In 2000, only 5,683 Malay individuals had university degrees—2,774 males and 2,908 females[4]. This was only 2 percent of the Malay population of 285,701. The proportion had increased from 0.2 percent for Malays in 1980, but remained far smaller than the 12.6 percent of Chinese or 16.5 percent of Indians who had attained university degrees. In addition, occupational status also varies between groups—according to census data, the Chinese are more likely to be employers or "own account workers," followed by Indians and then Malays. In 2000, among resident working persons aged 15 years and over, 2,535 Malay individuals were employers or "own account workers," representing 5.6 percent of the Malay population of 169,964, as compared to 15.4 percent of the Chinese or the 10.7 percent of Indians.

Population control and economic development

This section retraces important steps the Singaporean state has taken in its pursuit of economic development.

Table 3.7 Employment and education by gender (1965–2009)

Year	*Literacy rate (percent)*		*Combined gross enrolment ratio (percent)*		*Mean years of schooling*		*Labour force participation rate (percent of population aged 15 and over)*		*Working persons aged 15 and over (percent of total)*		*Professional, managerial, technical workers (percent of workforce)*	
	Male	*Female*	*Male*	*Female*	*Male*	*Female*	*Male*	*Female*	*Male*	*Female*	*Male*	*Female*
1965	76.4	42.6	74.1	64.8	n.a.	n.a.	80	24.2	78.8	21.2	n.a.	n.a.
1970	83	54.3	68.5	62.6	n.a.	n.a.	81.2	28.2	76.5	23.5	9	14.6
1975	87.2	64.7	66.6	63.1	n.a.	n.a.	79.3	34.9	70.5	29.5	14.4	11.4
1980	91.4	73.1	67.6	65.9	5.6	3.7	80.8	43.8	65.4	34.6	19.6	14.3
1985	93.2	78	76.6	74.4	6.5	4.9	n.a.	n.a.	n.a.	n.a.	n.a.	n.a.
1990	95.1	83	81	78.4	7.3	5.9	77.5	48.8	61.5	38.5	29.1	23.6
1995	95.8	85.8	86.9	83.5	8.4	7.2	77.2	46.8	62.1	37.9	38	31.9
2000	96.6	88.6	89.1	85.8	9.2	8.1	76.6	50.2	60	40	44.9	41.5
2005	97.3	91.1	94.3	93.1	9.9	8.8	74.4	52	58.3	41.7	45.5	43.9
2006	97.4	91.6	95.1	95	9.9	8.7	76.2	54.3	57.7	42.3	49.2	44
2007	97.6	92.1	95.9	96.4	9.9	8.8	76.5	54.3	57.5	42.5	50.3	47
2008	97.7	92.7	96	97.1	10.2	9.1	76.1	55.6	56.9	43.1	52.9	48.6
2009	97.9	93.3	96.3	96.4	10.3	9.2	76.3	55.2	57	43	53.1	50.6

Source:
Singapore Department of Statistics (2011e).

The Family Planning Association period (1949–1965)

The government's efforts concerning population management began with a rather modest private program, with some financial support from the British colonial government, as early as 1949. Specifically, as Saw (1980: 32) noted, during the post-WWII period:

> Apart from housing and educational problems, the government was confronted with the problem of feeding a large number of undernourished persons, especially children roaming the streets, because of rampant food shortages. The Social Welfare Department set up numerous centers to feed the hungry children, but it soon become apparent to the group of voluntary workers assisting in this scheme that, instead of feeding the children, the parents should be given family planning advice to plan their family size according to their means . . . A group of doctors, social workers and other interested individuals held a public meeting on 22 July 1949 to form the Family Planning Association (FPA) with the immediate aim of setting up clinics.

When Singapore became an independent nation in 1965, family planning activities conducted by the FPA were transferred to the new government's Health Ministry. As Suarez (2009: 17) pointed out:

> without access to the [Malaysian] Federation's market, import-substitution industrialization collapsed. The PAP government then decided to switch to export-oriented industrialization. One important aspect of this new strategy was dealing with uncompetitive labor costs . . . The government announced that it was doubling its population control efforts via fertility policies.

Anti-natalist period (1966–1983)

The Singapore Family Planning and Population Board

The Singapore Family Planning and Population Board Act was passed in 1965, and the Singapore Family Planning and Population Board (SFPPB) was established in 1966. The then Minister for Health, Dr. Yong Nyuk Lin, made the following remark during SFPPB's inaugural ceremony:

> Singapore, as we all know, is a very overcrowded little island of nearly 2 million people living in an area of just over 2 hundred square miles or a density of population around 8,000 people per square mile. Family planning is therefore a matter of national importance and indeed, one of urgency for us. Our best chances for survival in an independent Singapore is stress on quality and not quantity.
>
> (cited in Saw 2005: 25)

Population control efforts were aimed at reducing fertility rates to the replacement level as soon as possible. The Voluntary Sterilization Act was passed in 1969, and later repealed by the Voluntary Sterilization Act 1974, which made sterilization obtainable upon request and deemed it a private decision between applicants and doctors approving the procedure. The Abortion Act 1969 legalized induced abortion, and in 1974 abortion on demand was granted. Kee and Saw (1975: 109) reported:

> during 1966–1973, about 211,073 married women aged 15–44 (about 83 percent of all married women aged 15–44 in Singapore) were recorded as participants in the program; and 14,012 legal abortions, 23,445 female sterilizations, and 874 vasectomies were performed in government hospitals under the provision of Abortion Act of 1969 and the Voluntary Sterilization Act of 1969.

More importantly, additional policy measures were introduced to discourage large families. As Kirk (1980: vi) commented, "in the early 1970s Singapore embarked on a programme of incentives and disincentives . . . that is unique in the Third World and exceeded only by measures taken in the People's Republic of China." Indeed, the nation's first Prime Minister Lee Kuan Yew hinted at the forthcoming changes as early as his National Day message on 9 August 1965:

> We have to revise all our social values so that no one is required to have a large family in order to qualify for a Housing Board flat, for social relief and so on. Today, strange as it may seem, we are giving priority to people with large families, thereby encouraging people to have large families. This requires a revamping of all our social services, free primary schools, free hospitals and free maternity clinics regardless of how large the family is and the bigger social allowance given to the bigger families.

By August 1972 the government had announced the introduction of new incentives and disincentives (Saw 1980: 117). These measures included:

1. Reduction of income tax relief to cover three children only;
2. Lower priority for choice of primary school admission for children of fourth birth order and above;
3. An increase in delivery fees, with higher fees for children of higher birth order;
4. Elimination of priority for large families in the allocation of state-subsidized housing; and
5. Limitation of paid maternity leave to cover two children only.

The then Minister for Finance, Dr. Hon Sui Sen, explained in 1974:

> It is within the context of *total development* that the Singapore Government adopts a population policy to achieve zero population growth as soon as possible.
>
> (quoted in Saw 2005: 26, my emphasis).

Finally, as Kee and Loh (1974: 164) reported:

> The SFPPB in 1973 established [a] permanent liaison with all government ministries and statutory boards and many community organizations, trade unions, and voluntary and private agencies . . . Family planning and population subjects were included in the teacher training curriculum of the Institute of Education and in the regular courses of the Armed Forces. Population education was introduced into primary and secondary schools in 1973. During the year various groups, including social workers, medical students, doctors, nurses, community leaders, and labor and management personnel in the industries, held seminars to identify their roles in the national effort to limit population growth. At the same time, mass-media publicity was provided through the press, radio, television, cinemas, and exhibitions, while face-to-face motivation continued at the clinics, maternity wards, and homes.

In short, not only family planning programs such as contraception, abortion and sterilization, supplementary social disincentives, but also the intensive and comprehensive publicity and education efforts were all in place to encourage families to "stop at two (children)" during the anti-natalist period. As we shall see in later chapters, this contrasts sharply with the education and publicity efforts during the pronatalist period.

Kee and Loh (1974) analyzed the First National Survey on Family Planning in Singapore—Singapore's version of the Knowledge, Attitude and Practice (KAP) of family planning survey—conducted in 1973, and found that:

> 92 percent [of respondents] can name the higher delivery fees as one of the social disincentives. A lower proportion [i.e., 81 percent] is able to name maternity leave, perhaps because those who do not work would not be affected. Income tax relief for children is probably more familiar to the men.

Kee and Saw (1975) also analyzed the survey and found that "married women have a good knowledge of family planning methods. Ninety-eight percent have heard of at least one method, and 88 percent know how to use at least one method." More importantly, "around 75 percent of the married women are aware that the government recommends that every married couple in Singapore have no more than two children."

The total fertility rate reached 2.08, the replacement level, in 1975. As Wong and Yeoh (2003: 8) point out, "this watershed in Singapore's demographic history has been attributed to the combination of a number of factors rather than just the Old Population Policy [i.e., aforementioned anti-natalist policies] alone."

Intervening years (1984–1986)

The years 1983–1986 tend to be seen as the "eugenic phase" of Singapore's development. Saw suggested, "the year 1984 was the start of a new phase in the demographic history of Singapore[;] for the first time changes to the population control programme were designed to influence the *qualitative* aspect of the population." Key provisions included the following (Saw 1990):

1. Enhanced child relief for specially-educated women (at least five passes at Ordinary Level in the General Certificate of Education examination) to 5 percent of their earned income for the first child, 10 percent for the second child, and 15 percent for the third child, with, however, $10,000 as the maximum limit they can claim for each child.
2. Higher priority for choice of primary school admission for children of better-educated mothers (as noted in Chapter 2, the Graduate-Mother Priority Scheme was introduced in 1984 and withdrawn in 1985).
3. Mothers in all four classes pay the same hospital accouchement fees for fifth and subsequent children (a change from the old system which charged lower fees for the lower classes).
4. Sterilization cash incentive—the government offered a $10,000 cash grant through the women's Central Provident Fund (CPF) account under the following conditions: The mother must be under 30 years and be sterilized after the first or second child; neither parent should have any GCE Ordinary Level passes, combined monthly family income must not exceed $1,500; both parents must be Singaporean Citizens or permanent residents; should the mother produce another child, she must repay the $10,000 plus 10 percent compound interest per year; and neither the wife nor the husband must be earning more than $750 per month.
5. Graduate marriage matchmaking: The Social Development Unit (SDU) was established in 1984 to "provide matchmaking services to single graduate officers in government ministries, statutory boards, and government-owned companies."

Pronatalist period (1987–present)

Former Prime Minister Goh Chok Tong justified the shift to a pronatalist policy in his National Day Rally speech in 1986:

> the constraint of physical resources is not as difficult to overcome as the human resource problem . . . Put simply, there will not be enough young men to defend the country . . . What I am talking about is our ability to defend ourselves in the future.
>
> (cited by Wong and Yeoh 2003: 12)

Wong and Yeoh further note that:

> the new policy approach attempted to avoid the elitist tone of the eugenics era by setting a new "criterion" of "affordability." . . . It was based on the idea that people without secondary education could make up for their lack of education with "diligence, hard work, special talents, and skills."
>
> (ibid.)

As elaborated in Chapter 2, pronatalist policy measures—cash benefits (i.e., the Baby Bonus Scheme), income tax relief, tax rebates, childcare subsidies, use of Medisave accounts, lower maid levies, grandparent caregiver relief, priority in primary school registration, public sector flexible work, the five-day workweek, public sector leave, third child maternity leave, paid maternity leave, paid childcare leave, unpaid childcare leave, equal medical benefits, the Work-Life Works! Fund, public housing provisions, maternity leave protection, fertility treatment, and Social Development Units that provide matchmaking services—have become more comprehensive since 1987.

In addition, in the pronatalist context, in 1987 the government introduced "compulsory counselling" before abortion. However, as Saw (2007: 199) explained:

> this compulsory counselling, to be provided by doctors authorized to perform abortions in government and private hospitals, is applicable to only women with at least one or two children and with at least some secondary education. Hopefully, this counselling will provide all the essential facts concerning abortion to the women to give them a chance to change their mind and to proceed with the pregnancy.

In a similar fashion, while the government gave incentives during the anti-natalist phase for married women and men to undergo sterilization (for example, public sector employees were given one week's unrecorded leave immediately after undergoing tubal ligation or vasectomy), Saw (2007:204) noted the following:

> With effect from 1 April 1987, this one-week recorded leave was cancelled for those with one or more passes at Ordinary Level in the GCE examination, regardless of how many children they have. The intention of this change was to discourage government employees, *except the lowly-educated ones*, from going to sterilization and hence to continue to produce children in the future. There was also the old antinatalist policy intended to encourage women or their husbands to undergo sterilization by offering them lower accouchement fees in government hospitals. For B2 and C Class wards, the fees would be waived if the woman patient or her husband underwent sterilization within six weeks of the delivery of the baby. A modification of this scheme was put into effect on 1 April 1987 when the woman warded in these lower wards could only have the fees waived if she or her husband went for the sterilization operation after having the third of higher order births. The change is meant to stop discouraging couples with only one or two children from having more children.

The general abortion rate was 4.2 percent in 1970, then rose to peak at 31 percent in 1985 and declined to 12 percent in 2006 (ibid.: 200). In a similar fashion, the sterilization rate was 5.3 percent in 1970, peaked at 18.8 percent in 1976, and then decreased to 3.7 percent in 2005.

The National Population and Talent Division

While the SFPPB organized family planning services during the anti-natalist period, state policies proceeded without a central organizing body during the pronatalist period. Most recently, however, a national population management authority, the National Population Secretariat (NPS), was established in the Prime Minister's Office, in 2006. It was entrusted to:

> guide and coordinate whole-of-government efforts in the implementation of national population policies and programmes. It also provides secretariat support to the National Population Committee (NPC) chaired by the Deputy Prime Minister and Minister for Home Affairs Mr. Wong Kan Seng. The role of the NPC is to tackle the complex population challenge which requires planning and coordination at the highest level.
>
> (www.nptd.gov.sg)

The NPC was renamed the National Population and Talent Division (NPTD) in January 2011, and made responsible for (a) population augmentation; (b) supporting marriage and parenthood; (c) talent attraction and retention; (d) immigration, naturalization, and integration of newcomers; and (e) engaging overseas Singaporeans. As Liu (2011: 6) suggested, "although the Singapore government's foreign talents policy initiative did not aim at any particular ethnic sector, due to its migration history and geographical proximity, Chian became a main source of emigration." The organizational chart for the NPTD is shown in Figure 3.1.

Molding productive citizens

Singapore, like other "tiger economies" (Hong Kong, South Korea, and Taiwan), has been lauded for being able to sustain "a high-growth economy and a low social

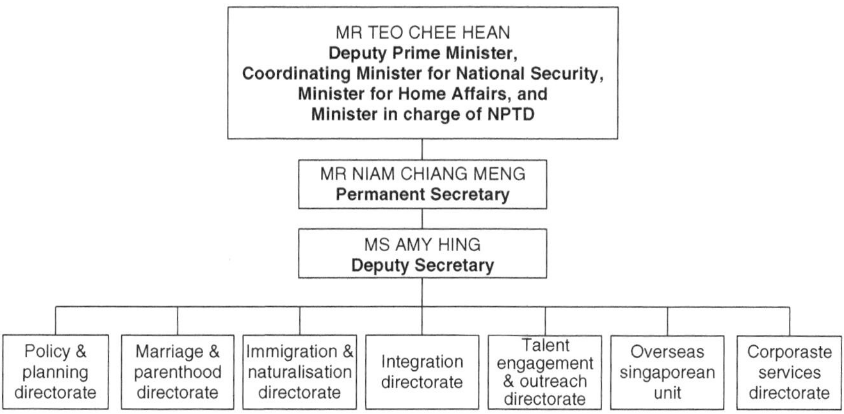

Figure 3.1 The National Population and Talent Division organizational chart

Source: National Population and Talent Division (2011b).

expenditure regime" (Jacobs 2000). Its achievements offer compelling evidence for an alternative model of economic development and social provision. "Selective" social provision underlies such success—the state provides welfare primarily to enable citizens to participate in paid employment, most notably through education. Moreover, social policies are mechanisms to encourage "self-reliance" and intra-familial support, mainly through the institution of the CPF. Finally, economically productive and responsible citizens are rewarded with state-subsidized and managed housing provisions. Moreover, as we shall see in the following chapters, the logic of "productivism" underlies not only economic production but also social reproduction of the nation. In sharp contrast to the observation that "the state will come to rescue those who are proven least able to help themselves" in social welfare provisions (Lee 2007: xv), however, we will see that "the state rewards those who are proven most economically able to help themselves" through the provision of pronatalist incentives. In short, the central concern that has shaped the Singaporean government's policies in social provisions and population policies has been molding "productive" citizens; the ideal citizen in the eyes of the state is an "economically" productive one.

4 Class-differentiated pronatalism

> The law, in its majestic equality, forbids rich and poor alike to sleep under bridges, to beg in the streets, and to steal their bread.
>
> Anatole France, 1894, *Le Lys Rouge*

In the public sphere, who is the ideal citizen? How is this ideal codified into public policy? Who is best informed about pronatalist financial incentives? In this chapter, I attempt to answer these questions. In their ground-breaking and now-classic paper on how decisions are made in uncertain situations, Tversky and Kahneman (1981) challenged the classical model of rational choice and presented the compelling case of "prospect theory." They showed how "variations in the framing of acts, contingencies, and outcomes" cause decision-making behavior to deviate from the expected utility theory. As the authors noted: "We use the term 'decision frame' to refer to the decision-maker's conception of the acts, outcomes, and contingencies associated with a particular choice" (1981: 453). In short, analysis of framing can help us better understand factors shaping the decision-making outcome. Below, I discuss how citizens perceive and respond to pronatalist incentives in terms of three main findings regarding, first, the predominant frame of childbearing decision-making that shapes policy effectiveness; second, communication and knowledge of government policies; and third, perceived class bias in existing economic incentives.

The predominant context of childbearing decision making

The first recurring response to government policies is the explicit recognition that Singapore is an expensive place to raise children. This constitutes the frame within which citizens consider whether government policies encourage them to have more children. Ninety-six of the 165 individual interviewees mentioned the high and rising cost of living in Singapore as a concern. More importantly, and interestingly, as Table 4.1 shows, those respondents who mentioned the rising cost of living tended to have reservations concerning the effectiveness of financial incentives in their responses to the following survey question: "Is the government policy making it easier financially for people to have more children?" Some straightforwardly said that the government subsidies had not made it financially easier to have children.

Table 4.1 Cost of Living and the respondents' perceptions toward financial incentives

Perceptions of the effectiveness of government's financial incentives	*Mentioned cost of living as a concern*	
	No, did not mention	*Yes, cost of living a concern*
Total	69 (100%)	96 (100%)
Unaware	11 (15.9%)	7 (7.3%)
Negative	23 (33.3%)	42 (43.8%)
Mixed, with reservations	18 (26.1%)	37 (38.5%)
Positive	17 (24.6%)	10 (10.4%)

Note N=165.

In contrast, those who did not mention such concerns tended to respond to the question positively.

Thus, on the one hand, citizens express appreciation for the Baby Bonus scheme; on the other hand, they give reasons for why the incentive amount is insufficient—a phenomenon similar to what Krugman described as "too little of a good thing" when analyzing the American Recovery and Reinvestment Act (Krugman 2009). For instance, Mrs. Ang (Chinese, monthly household income S$6,000–6,999) is 46 years old and has a son and a daughter. When asked to identify which policies were working to encourage childbearing and child rearing, she emphasized that the policies "all work," but then she went on to say: "They work, but just help a bit . . . Because the inflation and the standard of living is much greater than the help provided by these policies, you see."

Similarly, even though her husband "wants one football team," 33-year-old Mrs. Yatim (Malay, S$3,000–3,999) said, "two is just nice, one girl and one boy is just nice for me." She added, "The cost of bringing up children in Singapore is too high . . . And the medical fees [and] whatever things. Even your daily necessities for the kids, their education, you know."

It is not merely the increase in general living expenses, but also specific and immediate costs for newborns—for example diapers, milk, and vaccinations—that discourage more births. Mr. and Mrs. Balasingam (Indian, S$4,000–4,999), both 34 years old, with two children and a monthly household income of S$4,000–4,999 explained why the S$6,000 baby bonus subsidy for a third child was not attractive:

MR. BALASINGAM: So after we have our third child they [the government] give us S$6,000 cash, OK. Does the government know how much it costs when a baby is just born?

MRS. BALASINGAM: First year [the baby bonus is] already exhausted. Pampers . . . napkins . . . do you know a bottle of soap that we use to wash the baby's milk bottle, it's about S$14–15 a bottle and it lasts about a week and a half. OK. And you have so many other things to buy. All this requires cash, not to forget you need someone to help with the babysitting, certain kinds of food, children's vaccination, and there are a lot of nitty-gritties which are not calculated. You bring your child to a clinic, [and] you got to take a cab back if it's newborn. All these are also costs.

In other words, seen through a frame of rising prices of goods and services, the government's baby bonus subsidy is perceived and experienced as a form of reimbursement or compensation, rather than an extra benefit for having a child. As noted above, approximately two-thirds of the 165 interviewees mentioned cost of living as a concern. Further data analysis suggests that married respondents in upper-income households are *more* likely to bring up the issue of cost of living than their counterparts in middle- and lower-income households; this is true even though lower-income families are reported to be most affected by inflation:

> Families with monthly household income [in] the bottom 20 per cent face a 7.4 per cent . . . inflation rate, which is above the 7.1 per cent national average. The top 20 per cent and the rest middle-income all face [a] 6.9 per cent . . . inflation rate.
>
> (Hu 2008: A1)

Moreover, as shown in Table 4.2, the inflation rate increased by more than four percent between November 2006 and November 2007. At the same time, as shown in Table 4.3, the real annual change in average monthly household income for the bottom 20 percent is less than 4 percent. In other words, the increase in cost of living exceeds the increase in income, especially for households earning below S$3,000 a month.

Below, I elaborate on the three specific types of subsidies—education, healthcare, and housing—that respondents highlighted in their answers to the following open-ended questions:

- If you are deciding whether to have a child, is there anything the government can do that will help you decide?
- What needs to be done by the government in terms of policies to encourage people to have more children?
- What is it that you need in order to have the number of children you want?

Education

Citizens acknowledged that primary and secondary school education had been heavily subsidized by the state in Singapore. But they then listed items that they still had to pay for out of their own pockets, such as school fees, books, assignment booklets, transportation, tuition, and extracurricular activities. Thus, they perceived

Table 4.2 Inflation (January 2007–August 2008)

Month/year	*Consumer Price Index (annual change)*
January '07	0.2
February '07	0.6
March '07	0.7
April '07	0.6
May '07	1.0
June '07	1.3
July '07	2.6
August '07	2.9
September '07	2.7
October '07	3.6
November '07	4.2
December '07	4.4
January '08	6.6
February '08	6.5
March '08	6.7
April '08	7.5
May '08	7.5
June '08	7.5
July '08	6.5
August '08	6.4

Source: Singapore Department of Statistics, *Singapore Consumer Price Index*, various years.

Table 4.3 Average earned monthly household income

Decile	*2006 (S$)*	*2007 (S$)*	*2008 (S$)*	*Real annual change (percent)*		
				2006	*2007*	*2008*
Total	6,280	6,890	7,750	2.7	7.5	5.7
1st–10th	1,170	1,220	1,310	0.0	2.5	0.1
11th–20th	2,130	2,240	2,480	1.1	3.0	3.2
21st–30th	2,880	3,040	3,430	1.0	3.4	6.0
31st–40th	3,660	3,970	4,430	0.6	6.4	4.7
41st–50th	4,490	4,900	5,460	0.2	7.2	4.6
51st–60th	5,480	5,880	6,730	2.7	5.3	7.5
61st–70th	6,460	7,140	8,040	–1.2	8.4	5.8
71st–80th	8,010	8,730	9,720	3.1	6.8	4.7
81st–90th	10,110	11,330	12,910	2.7	9.6	7.6
91st–100th	18,410	20,440	23,020	6.4	8.6	6.3

Source: Singapore Department of Statistics (2009b).

that overall expenditures remained too high for them to consider having another child. They wanted more state subsidies—63 of the 165 individual interviewees (38 percent) wanted educational subsidies, but respondents in upper-income households (with monthly household incomes exceeding S$8,000) were less likely to want such subsidies than their counterparts in lower- and middle-income households, as shown in Table 4.4. That said, more than one-third of respondents in each income bracket wanted educational subsidies.

Moreover, a notable number of interviewees suggested "free education" for citizens—that is elimination of the nominal school fees that they were paying especially since primary school education is compulsory. These fees were perceived as a burden that the government should bear as a matter of principle, as argued by Mr. Rahimi (Malay, age 27, S$3,000–3,999):

MR. RAHIMI: We have lots of government schools, but I don't see the need to have to pay fees for government schools. Can't they just subsidize across the board? Compulsory education for everybody so you shouldn't need to pay school fees. Across the board, across all races.

MODERATOR: How much are school fees?

MR. RAHIMI: S$20-plus a month for a child, about there. So even S$20–30, you add up for a year it's already 30 times 12, S$400 to S$500-plus. So imagine, ease off all these on education because it's already a government school. And you even pay taxes. Pay income tax to finance schools. So why not make education free? Like how other countries are doing it? Public schools are free unless you choose to go to a private school.

The Singapore government's stance on compulsory education and the policy of free public education for citizens in countries such as Australia—as one interviewee pointed out, "As long as you're a citizen, they provide this for you"—were mentioned repeatedly by other interviewees across the income strata.[1] Thus, interviewees expressed a strong desire for free education as a public good and perhaps even a

Table 4.4 Requests for more education subsidies by the respondents' monthly household income

	Monthly household income (S$)			
	Below 3000	*3000–7999*	*8000 and above*	*Total*
Total	40 (100%)	85 (100%)	38 (100%)	163 (100%)
No comments	22 (55.0%)	53 (62.4%)	25 (65.8%)	100 (61.3%)
More subsidies	18 (45.0%)	32 (37.6%)	13 (34.2%)	63 (38.7%)

Note N=163.

social right for citizens, although their remarks were not couched explicitly in these terms.

Respondents placed a great emphasis on education, including preschool and tertiary education. The former provides a foundation for primary and secondary schooling, while the latter is seen as a vehicle for upward mobility. In terms of preschool education, there are two kinds of service providers: PAP (People's Action Party) Community Foundation kindergartens and private kindergartens. In 2008, a typical PAP kindergarten charged about S$100 a month for a half-day program covering five mornings a week, while fees for private kindergartens varied from several hundred dollars to more than S$1,000 per month for full-day programs. As noted in Chapter 2, the government provides working mothers with a monthly infant-care (18 months to 2 years old) subsidy capped at S$600 per child, and a childcare subsidy capped at S$300 per child. The maximum infant-care and child-care subsidy for non-working mothers is S$150 per child.

Even with state subsidies, parents in lower-middle-income families found preschool "very expensive" because there are additional costs associated with going to preschool, such as bus fares. Mrs. Ibrahim (Malay, age 49, S$3,000–3,999) and Mr. Idris (Malay, age 40, S$3,000–3,999), for instance, talked about their son's preschool expenditures:

MRS. IBRAHIM: Preschool is the school fees and the transport. Very expensive. Very, very expensive.

MR. IDRIS: Very expensive.

MODERATOR: How expensive?

MRS. IBRAHIM: If kindergarten, about S$120 per month. If you have to send him by transport, it's about, just nearby, a few bus stop away only, about S$100 . . .

Parents in higher-income families were also discouraged by school fees because they anticipate sending their child(ren) to private kindergartens.[2] As Mr. Lee (Chinese, five-room HDB apartment, S$10,000 and over) explained:

> Do you have enough income to put them into preschool or nurseries, you know, because the private ones cost like S$600–700 a month, and that's only the fee. Enrichment classes and all those sort of stuff, it's an additional cost . . .

If parents in upper-income families were concerned about education expenses in their childbearing decisions, parents in lower-middle-income families were worried about paying tertiary school fees, even after receiving government grants. As Mr. Rahimi (Malay, age 27, S$3,000–3,999) and his sister Jamilah pointed out:

MR. RAHIMI: Education. It's very big because now you can't survive at [GCE] O-Levels. Even if you get [GCE] A-Level, a diploma, it's not enough, you still need to keep going up. Even a degree is not sufficient, and everyone is like doctors, doctors, professors, professors, doctors, anyway in order to be someone.

For every semester [six months] . . . after [government] grants, it's S$1,000. That's minimum. So S$1,000 [per semester] over a three-year period is about S$6,000. And that is for now up to a poly [polytechnic] level. Nowadays for poly, you also can't survive. You have to upgrade because nowadays people are going to [get university] degrees.

JAMILAH: S$6,000 [per year for a university degree]. So if you take four years would be about S$24,000.

Respondents recognized that university education was heavily subsidized by the state, but as Mr. and Mrs. Krishnamurthy (Indian, in their mid-50s, private property, S$3,000–3,999) pointed out, "Even though it is heavily subsidized, it is not enough. Quite a lot of money we have to spend for university and all." In the following conversation with Mr. and Mrs. Goh (Chinese, four-room HDB apartment, S$4,000–4,999) and their friends Mr. and Mrs. Tay (Chinese, five-room HDB apartment, S$4,000–4,999), Mr. Goh proclaimed, "It's tertiary [education tuition] that will kill":

MR. GOH: I think tertiary education subsidies would be a major draw. Because her [referring to his daughter attending a local university] fees is like S$6,000 a year, which translates to about S$500 a month, and expenses is like another S$500–600 a month, so that works out to about S$1,200 average per month, so where are we going to get money? Eventually, I hope the child will be getting tertiary education. So I have to anticipate, like now I give birth to a child. Yes, primary and secondary education is not so expensive. Somehow we'll make ends meet, but it's tertiary [education] that will kill. Actually, it has been said that it's heavily subsidized, but still it's a big expense in the home.

MR. TAY: This is a major thing. Two or three of my friends, they study up till A-Level [i.e., the Singapore-Cambridge General Certificate of Education Advanced Level, called GCE A-Level], cannot afford, got to help the family, so they got to work two to three years, then they go study their own degree course.

Mr. Goh also commented on the CPF education scheme:

> So the policies for this thing is that yes, you can take a loan from CPF. It's an interest-free loan, which is very good . . . It's still a loan, so it translates into somebody has got to pay the loan. So the government can come in. Scholars will surely get the scholarship, subsidies, and all that, but what about the non-scholars? The bulk of them is non-scholars.

In sum, although interviewees were positive about pronatalist financial incentives, they said they would appreciate considerably larger and more long-term subsidies in education. Citizens in lower- and even middle-income households are hurt by rising costs and struggling to make ends meet, while citizens in higher-income households are also "on a budget," as they have higher expectations for their children. Substantial state provisions would help to make childrearing more affordable and imaginable.

Healthcare

Singaporean government-subsidized healthcare care is provided by public hospitals and neighborhood polyclinics, which are utilized by citizens who cannot afford the higher healthcare costs of the private sector. In addition, as noted in Chapter 3, payment for certain categories of medical care can be drawn from citizens' accumulated CPF savings through a Medisave account (for non-employed immediate relatives as well as for themselves).

However, lower- and middle-income families find it difficult to cope with high prescription costs, which can run into hundreds of dollars, even under the public healthcare system. 51 of the 165 individual interviewees (approximately 30 percent) wanted more healthcare subsidies. As shown in Table 4.5, in each income bracket, about 30 percent of respondents indicated that more healthcare subsidies would be conducive to childbearing.

In addition, long queues for consultation are discouraging, as the following conversation with Mr. Ibrahim (Malay, age 52) and Mrs. Ibrahim (Malay, age 49, S$3,000–3,999) and Mr. Idris (Malay, age 40) and Mrs. Idris (Malay, age 42, S$3,000–3,999) indicated:

MRS. IBRAHIM: Health expenses also increased. If the children [get] sick, like HFMD [i.e., hand, foot, and mouth disease], that kind of thing, then [the child has to] stay in hospital. I mean hospitalized, then go for check-up. Now, as you know, the expenses are very high. When they refer you to an A&E [accident and emergency], now you have to pay S$70; and [you] cannot use Medisave. If referred from polyclinics, it's cheaper. I think S$5 or S$10 [cheaper] than referred by private clinic. If you go to polyclinic, you queue. Can be one to two [hours], two [hours]-plus . . .

Table 4.5 Requests for more health subsidies by the respondents' monthly household income

	Monthly household income (S$)			
	Below 3,000	*3,000–7,999*	*8,000 and above*	*Total*
Total	40 (100%)	85 (100%)	38 (100%)	163 (100%)
No comments	28 (70.0%)	59 (69.4%)	26 (68.4%)	113 (69.3%)
More subsidies	12 (30.0%)	26 (30.6%)	12 (31.6%)	50 (30.7%)

Note N=163.

Long queues at polyclinics are generally seen as problematic, but especially for parents with young children, as the following conversation with Mrs. Visvanathan (Indian, age 48, S$1,000–1,999) and Mrs. Nair (Indian, age 51, S$5,000–5,999) suggests. Thus, citizens may turn to care provided by neighborhood general practitioners, who charge higher fees:

MRS. NAIR: The medical expense here is quite expensive.

MODERATOR: How expensive?

MRS. NAIR: Oh, of course definitely at the minimum is S$32. Any GP [general practitioner] . . . In case of an emergency, you cannot go to the polyclinic and wait so long. Especially when they are young, you know, because I face this problem, that's why I am telling. The medical expense is quite high, S$32 or S$38.60 sometimes. Then you want to book an X-ray or blood test, then everything comes up to two hundred or three hundred. They [the state] should subsidize.

Similar to Mrs. Nair's point that unforeseen complications engender higher costs, Mr. and Mrs. Balasingam, mentioned earlier, provided another example of how healthcare costs increase because young children tend to catch one another's illnesses:

MRS. BALASINGAM: People creating our policies should be in our shoes. . . . It's very easy to sit in a room and come up with plans very nicely . . . and it looks very nice on paper. Wow, S$6,000. I mean, when you have three kids, four kids, and when one falls sick, all fall sick. And there is no way we can waive off the consultation fees. I think the doctor just saw dollar signs. The whole family is here. It's to the point that I share the medicine with my kids. That's not the way, right? I should not even worry about medicine.

MR. BALASINGAM: That one week we go down to the doctor is about [cost us] S$200 cash. We're not talking about the cash amount here; we're talking about policy, education, and health. Can you [the state] provide free health coverage for my child until he goes to National Service or tertiary education? . . . At the polyclinic. It doesn't have to be at the private hospital. That means I bring my child to the polyclinic . . . There are a lot of people who don't have a high income, you know.

Among higher-income families, there is a willingness to turn to private-sector healthcare providers, who are perceived as offering better service. However, even with their significantly higher incomes, in seeking better healthcare these families too want more government subsidies. For example, one pronatalist measure that the Singapore government has adopted since 1987, and has continued to refine, allows usage of the CPF Medisave account for childbearing purposes. However, use of the Medisave account is perceived as "still using our own money," and so does not satisfy citizens' desires for more state-provided subsidies. This is illustrated in the following focus group discussion with Mr. and Mrs. Lee, also cited above, who held their infant during the interview:

MODERATOR: If the government really wants to help . . .

MR. LEE: Up-front cost hospitalization, delivery charges. We went to Mount Alvernia [hospital], she [referring to Mrs. Lee] did a caesarean, more than S$7,000 . . . The gynecological fees and everything, so that up-front [subsidies] would definitely be helpful.

MRS. LEE: That's already up-front, not to mention actually the nine months you are carrying the baby to see the gynecologist. The medical check-ups and everything.

MODERATOR: So how did you finance those?

MRS. LEE: Through our own means. Through our own money. But I think they do give. Apparently they are saying you can still claim your [CPF] Medisave. But it's your own money. They [the government] allow, but it's still your own money.

Similarly, the S$3,000 Baby Bonus cash incentive is perceived as insufficient. Mr. Khaw pointed out that delivery and hospitalization expenditures are high at private hospitals:

MR. KHAW: Of course, the money [the subsidy] is there. But you're talking about S$3,000 over a period of eighteen months. Three thousand dollars barely covers. If let's say someone, for example, doesn't have the CPF, who's not working and doesn't have the CPF, cannot have Medisave coverage, he will have to fork out cash. For example, our stay at the Thomson Medical Centre amounted to almost S$8,000. So Medisave covered about almost S$5,000-odd, so we have to fork out another S$2,000-odd. Of course, you'll say, "It's because you chose Thomson Medical Centre [a private hospital]; who asked you to choose Thomson Medical Centre?" But you know, in terms of facilities and professionalism so far as other mothers have experienced, these are the recommended places.

In summary, citizens from all income strata want the state to provide more healthcare financial support for the making of future citizens, albeit with different rationales. On the one hand, citizens in lower-income households face a struggle with prescription fees and encounter long waits at government-subsidized polyclinics and find the situation particularly difficult with young children; and citizens in middle-income households are trying to pay overall higher fees at neighborhood clinics. On the other hand, citizens in higher-income households also spend large sums on healthcare, as they want to receive better treatment, particularly in private hospitals and medical centers.

Housing

The purchase of HDB apartments, as noted in Chapter 3, entails an initial cash deposit followed by monthly payments over a number of years—which, in the case of employed persons, can be drawn from CPF accounts and supplemented with bank loans, if necessary. Housing constitutes a sizable portion of cost of living, even for middle-income working couples. This is more so given that prices in the housing market (for both HDB and private homes) have increased dramatically over the years. 13 of the 165 interviewees (7.9 percent) perceived housing to be expensive and wanted more housing subsidies, and respondents belonging to upper-income households (with a monthly household income exceeding S$8,000) were more likely than their counterparts to express such desires—partly due to the state's rule that these high-income households are not allowed to purchase a HDB flat.

In a focus group interview with Mrs. Majid (Malay, age 28, S$5,000–5,999) and family members (Mrs. Majid's mother, Malay, age 52, below S$1,000; and Mrs. Majid's sister, Malay, age 22, university student), it was pointed out that, despite having a higher income than her mother, Mrs. Majid had to pay more for her four-room HDB apartment, priced at S$215,000, compared to her mother, who paid over five years for her five-room HDB apartment, priced at S$125,000. Moreover, Mrs. Majid reported that, with the housing loan and interest, the actual amount that she had to pay was nearly double what her mother paid, and she had to pay over a longer period of time.

MRS. MAJID'S SISTER: Yeah . . . in terms of housing, my mother wouldn't have to worry about it anymore after five years; [although] my sister has higher income, she has to pay for longer.

MRS. MAJID'S MOTHER: And you [referring to Mrs. Majid] have four-room flats only, not even five rooms. Mine is a five-room point block, the biggest [type of HDB] flat in Singapore. The most expensive flat. Point block, they call it. I bought that one, second buyer, S$125,000, and yet I [could] finish it [i.e., the full payment] in five years.

MRS. MAJID'S SISTER: S$125,000. But for her, how much is your flat?

MRS. MAJID: S$215,000.

MRS. MAJID'S SISTER: But, with the loan and everything, become what?

MRS. MAJID: Double. Almost double.

In what follows, I draw on the focus group discussion with Mr. and Mrs. Balasingam, the Indian couple mentioned earlier, and their friends Mr. Syed (Indian, age 27, S$3,000–3,999) and Mrs. Syed (Indian, age 30, S$3,000–3,999). Mrs. Syed offered another illustration of the financial burden involved in servicing an HDB loan over the long term, particularly for couples with modest incomes, who must also ensure that they remain continually employed to keep contributing to their CPF accounts.

MRS. SYED: For example, my mother-in-law's place, she bought a house for S$190–200,000, she pays S$330 through her CPF every month so it depletes her CPF, right? So when I look at her mortgage statement, the S$330 every month, almost S$180 goes into interest. There's a larger percentage going to interest rather than the principal. So she's going to spend twenty-five years

> paying S$330. In the end she pays a total of double the amount that she bought the house for.

In addition, parents who intended to have another child also anticipate the need to have more rooms. This is illustrated by Mr. Khaw (age 30) and Mrs. Khaw (age 28, S$7,000–7,999), a dual-income couple with a one-year-old son, Nicholas, who own a five-room HDB apartment Mr Khaw said:

> Having more children also means we need a bigger place. And I think maybe previously when our parents they lived in . . . I think that time it was much cheaper . . . They lived in kampong-type [village-type] of living. Wide space, and they all crammed together. . . . But now in our current kind of lifestyle, we don't sleep in squatters, three-layer beds . . . Right now we're concerned that next time we may want to get a bigger place so that the children can have their own rooms.

Similarly, Mr. Balasingam, introduced earlier, said:

> If you have four kids and a four-room flat, when they grow up, each one of them wants a room, Mummy and Daddy will sleep in the hall. It's all bread and butter issues. Nobody is asking for things over the moon.

What these accounts show is that even with the state-subsidized housing provisions, citizens in lower- and middle-income families find it difficult to acquire a roof over their head, a precondition for them to consider another child. In particular, they are discouraged by rising prices and the attendant longer period of housing loan payments. And if they use their CPF savings to pay for the loans, there are additional CPF interest payments. In contrast, the barrier for middle- and upper-income households is not so much the inability to pay but expectations of upgrading to a bigger apartment with a room for each child.

Communication and knowledge of government policies

The second consistent finding is that details of government policies are vague, unspecified, or simply unknown among citizens. Even for the better-publicized Baby Bonus scheme, only approximately one in five of the 165 respondents could provide details such as the bonus amount or the time frame of such benefits in their answers to the following list of survey questions:

- Was there anything the government did that helped you decide to have a child/children? (For married respondents);
- If you are deciding whether to have a child, is there anything the government can do that will help you decide? (For unmarried respondents);
- As far as you know, has the government done anything to help families in Singapore? If yes, can you please tell me what the Singapore government has

done? If no, what do you think needs to be done by the government to help families? (For all respondents); and

- As far as you know, is there any government policy that encourages people to have more children? If yes, can you please tell me what those policies are? Which policies do you think actually work? Among these policies, which one(s) do you think are not working? If no, what needs to be done by the government in terms of policies to encourage people to have more children?

In answering these questions, the majority (70 percent) of respondents either knew only catchphrases for the policies, without details, or were completely unaware of them (12 percent). Moreover, there is an inverse relationship between respondents' educational levels and understanding of such policies, as indicated in Table 4.6.

This finding of limited knowledge of pronatalist policies is consistent with Straughan, Chan, and Jones's 2009 study. The authors noted that:

> while almost 40 percent were well informed about the new family policies, it is interesting to note that almost a quarter had not heard about the new initiatives at all. Given the limited geographical expanse of this nation-state and the communication channels in place, this is indeed surprising.
>
> (p. 193)

Data in this study suggest that women with a lower educational level are especially poorly informed about the relevant policies.

In what follows, I report on an extensive focus group interview with 36-year-old Mazlan (Malay, polytechnic diploma, S$3,000–3,999) and his girlfriend Jamilah

Table 4.6 Respondents' educational attainment and knowledge about pronatalist financial incentives

Knowledge about pronatalist financial incentives	*Respondents' highest level of education*			
	Primary school	*Secondary and pre-university*	*University-educated*	*Total*
Total	3 (100%)	57 (100%)	105 (100%)	165 (100%)
Unaware	1 (33.3%)	8 (14.0%)	10 (9.5%)	19 (11.5%)
Keyword	2 (66.7%)	37 (64.9%)	78 (74.3%)	117 (70.9%)
Detail	0 0.0%	12 (21.1%)	17 (16.2%)	29 (17.6%)

Note N=165.

(Malay, other diploma, S$3,000–3,999), to illustrate how "word-of-mouth" dissemination may disadvantage respondents in less-educated households. When probed about the "lower maid levy" initiative, Mazlan showed no knowledge of the policy and its details, and asked, "Is it been published in the newspaper for all these?" Speaking for himself and his friends, he said:

> It's very hard for us even to take notice. Because some of them, my friends, they don't read newspaper daily. Like those from the lower income, even to buy the newspapers at 80 cents, 90 cents. For them, it is still a lot. I got a friend who earns a certain [low] amount. He doesn't know about all these things, about this baby bonus thing or whatever it is. So he came to know about it when he met the MP [member of parliament] to ask for help. The MP tell him about this.

When asked why his friend didn't know about the policies, Mazlan said:

> He doesn't because he don't read newspapers. I think he don't know how to read newspapers. The problem is, the word of mouth, the things have not been channeled all the way down . . . Actually he has three kids . . . He borrows from neighbors, relatives in order to survive on staple food, which eventually, all these things add up to this. So what I think is that he just seeks help from the MP and that is when he knows all these things.

It may not be surprising that there are citizens who cannot make ends meet and have to resort to loans and government subsidies; what this instance reveals is that these may also be citizens who lack knowledge about pronatalist policies. As Jamilah added:

> They are not informed of all these, I guess . . . It's not based on the policies that they want to have children. It's not by [due to] things that the government is doing. They decide they themselves want to start a family. But it's not possible, because it gets harder, and the thing is that they do not know about the policies, so it's not helping. They are struggling.

In the focus group interview with a dual-income, Chinese, married couple with a combined monthly household income of S$4,000–4,999, Mr. Khaw, a 30-year-old university graduate, told of the surprisingly low take-up rate of "free computers." This provides further illustration as to why it is difficult to disseminate information on policies among less-educated households:

> Even with all the [baby bonus] subsidies and all, some parents may not be aware that they can go, and these people who are not aware may not be educated people who can read what you give to them . . . brochures and all . . . I mean, I know because right now we have this funding to give to students with no computers a computer, and it's free. We give them forms and documents, but

> the take-up rate is low. Because these forms . . . so many words . . . given by the government. They can't read the forms. So they think that they have to pay for the computer, then they don't want it. You know, they don't understand. So we have to create ways where we actually invite them to come, and we explain to them verbally and let them know this is free. And then on the spot they go and . . . Then the take-up rate is more. It's definitely important to let the lower-income know, especially . . . The educated, if they are retrenched, they'll be able to understand these policies and all.

What the above exchange suggests is that policy information is not readily available to members of less-educated households, making policies less likely to form a basis for their decision making. The desire for the state to be more effective in communicating its policies is poignantly crystallized in the focus group discussion with a middle-income Chinese couple. Mr. Goh (age 44, university graduate, S$3,000–3,999) and Mrs. Goh (age 43, stay-at-home mother) have three daughters. Mr. Goh says:

> Correct me if I'm wrong. Our government way of doing things is like "I'm not going to spoon-feed you, to bring the money to your account per se. You have to come and find out and take whatever you need." I think this is more cost-effective, more cost-efficient, fair enough. So how am I going to know if you're not going to bring the information to me? After all, not many people are going to read and find out information, like say, if you're going to have a fourth child, you go and find out. But so tired, the whole day is enough. Ask me to find out more information? Oh please.

In other focus group discussions, respondents provided further insights into ways for the government to help raise awareness of pronatalist benefits. For example, while, at the moment, married couples tend to learn of such policies at the hospital, they would prefer to be informed at an earlier stage, such as at the gynecologists' clinic. Mr. Khaw explained:

> Generally, what happened is, I say prior to all these, we hear about it. So then we go online, check what baby bonus is all about. Then they have their website and we look through it. Then more information, actual information only came about at the hospitals, when the child was born, then suddenly there's this package given to us. [But] I think it would have been better if, for example, at the clinics, all the different gynecologists that we go, they already give us the advance preparation.
>
> [Moderator: Why?]
>
> Because at least during the whole nine-month process, at least we can start to understand the whole thing rather than at the registration; it's more or less like just filling in forms to get the money, more than what we are able to plan for. So that's why if you do it at a gynecologist, like prenatal stage, at least

> you know these are the things that are covered. By the time [of the baby's birth] I'll be busy and alone, she'd be bedridden. I'll also have to run around entertaining people who come and visit; then there's not really much chance for me to really look into it.

This idea of disseminating state pronatalist policies at the clinics was also suggested by Jamilah. She further suggested that "it should be made automatic":

> Only those who are educated and who know about it will apply for it. It should be made automatic. As in it's there, you want it, you take it. If you don't want it, you say you don't want, rather than you opt in to be in it. Make it automated, once you have a baby. Because [the baby] is registered already. So make it for this baby, and then send the information to the parents. If they do not want, they decline.

University students also suggested targeting younger adults. Indeed, respondents engaged in animated dialogues with each other and suggested specific ways of addressing the issue of information dissemination, such as posting information on residential buildings' notice boards, mailing pronatalist policy packages to newly-wed couples as "reading material," and having "a web page in the Registry of Marriage portal"—rather than publicizing it during the annual National Day Rally speech, which, according to Hui Ling (Chinese, S$2,000–2,999), "people hardly listen to."

Class differentiation in existing economic incentives

The third repeated finding concerning pronatalist financial incentives from this study is the perceived and experienced bias in existing economic incentives such as the dollar-for-dollar matching funds Children Development Accounts (CDA) and tax rebates.

Responses toward tax rebates

As Lin and Rantalaiho (2003) pointed out, tax rebates constitute the primary means through which the Singaporean government delivers its benefits. The majority of interviewees did not make evaluative comments about the government's tax rebates in their answers to survey questions listed earlier; indeed, only 13 out of 165 interviewees did (11 had positive comments, while 2 had negative comments). Such a number is certainly too small to draw any conclusive statements from. However, it is worth noting that, while only 1 in 5 of the 165 interviewees owned or resided in a private condominium or landed property, the ratio was 3 in 5 among respondents with positive comments on tax rebates. In other words, respondents from wealthier households disproportionately constituted those who praised tax rebates as a form of pronatalist financial subsidy in this sample.

This pattern also rings true for the focus group discussions, where married couples who responded positively to tax rebates tended to come from wealthier backgrounds. For instance, when I asked an upper-class Chinese couple with landed property, a combined monthly household income of more than S$10,000, and an only daughter, what policy initiatives were helpful, Mr. Owyong replied: "I would say only the income tax portion . . . yeah, the income tax's kind of relief that benefit the people having more than one kid or two kids."

This is similar to another focus group discussion with Mr. and Mrs. Lee, a married Chinese couple in their 30s living in a five-room HDB apartment with a combined monthly household income of more than S$10,000. When I asked "When you gave birth to the first child, what kind of policies were in place? What was your experience?" Mrs. Lee explained, "I guess it's only the income tax, I think. It's the child relief income tax." Mr. Lee followed up: "It's positive, but again it does not affect our decision to have kids."

As observed in focus group discussions, while respondents acknowledged that they benefited from tax rebates, they stressed that these were not the reason for them to have a first or additional child. However, tax rebates are materially irrelevant for childbearing and child-rearing dynamics in less-wealthy households, as illustrated in the following conversation with Mr. and Mrs. Chong, a Chinese couple in their 40s living in a three-room HDB flat and earning a combined monthly household income of S$2,000–2,999:

MRS. CHONG: This tax rebate program is only useful for people with higher pay. How much tax can be deducted from people of the middle class like us? Honestly speaking, they have not deducted a cent of tax for my employment of more than ten years, because there is nothing for them to deduct. The same goes for him [referring to Mr. Chong].

MR. CHONG: If our society continues to work this way, honestly speaking, the people will only make one move. It is to sell their houses and strike out for themselves new paths in another country. They will all migrate and leave Singapore if they manage to find a good place. There are many who [are] already doing this. They moved together and not singly . . . In the case where we wish to increase our population, regardless whether one is poor or rich, there can be a scheme where all the people can bring the child's birth certificate to claim the milk powder subsidized by the government. Whether the child needs two-and-a-half or three years of supply, purchase the milk powder with the birth certificate. It should be equal to all regardless of race. Education is free for all, be it Chinese and Malay. As long as you are Singapore citizen, it is free.

This theme is further illuminated by Mr. Balasingam, introduced earlier, who explained:

> Do you know how much you have to earn a month to be liable for tax? I think a yearly income of about S$22,000. S$20,000 to S$22,000 income for one person to be liable for income tax. I can tell you there are a lot of people out there who do not meet that criterion.

Indeed, Singapore residents have to earn an annual chargeable income of more than S$22,000 to be liable for tax (Inland Revenue Authority Singapore 2008). In other words, the average monthly income has to be S$1,833. According to the 2005 General Household Survey, 70 percent of the resident population has an average monthly per capita household income of only S$1,580, which means no tax and, therefore, no tax rebates. In short, respondents are able to articulate what they perceive to be a bias in the policies: private-property-owning citizens find the tax rebates helpful and beneficial; on the other hand, the scheme is immaterial for less-wealthy households.

Responses toward dollar-for-dollar Children Development Account

There are two components to the Baby Bonus scheme instituted in 2000. All parents, regardless of family size and income, receive lump-sum cash benefits of S$4,000 for a first and second child, and S$6,000 each for a third and fourth child. In addition, the Singaporean government provides a matching contribution for a child's Children Development Account (CDA). In 2008, the government announced that while a fifth child and beyond were not eligible for cash grants, the government would provide a matching contribution of up to S$18,000 for them.

The majority of the 165 individual female respondents did not make evaluative comments about the CDA; only 11 did (9 respondents had negative comments, while 2 had positive comments). Again, such numbers do not allow for any conclusive statements. However, it is worth noting that, among respondents who had negative comments, none had a monthly household income exceeding S$7,000, while the only two respondents who had positive comments did.

During focus group interviews with married couples who had used the CDA, it became clear that even respondents from middle-income households had difficulty saving and benefiting from the scheme. For example, in the interview with the Chinese couple introduced above, Mr. Khaw reported:

> The thing is, we have to fork out the S$3,000 first, then they'll match dollar-for-dollar. But if we are already in financial difficulty, it's very hard to cough out that S$3,000 for the government to match it dollar-for-dollar. So let's say I can only come out with S$500? Then effectively my Baby Bonus, so to speak, is S$1,000.

Other middle-class parents also articulated the way in which the CDA scheme hinges on their income level. When asked about the CDA account, Mrs. Balasingam showed that she understood it was a "dollar-to-dollar match." But her husband noted the following in response to her saying that they "don't have that extra money [that they] still have to put in [so that] the government would top it up":

> That's [CDA] not money in your pocket. So eventually I still have to come up with 50 percent. I take my cash, and I put it in the bank. The bank gets the money, the government tops it up. But until that money is exhausted, I can't

> take back 50 percent of my money . . . which means I'm still cash-poor . . . I have to still come up with the money at the beginning. What I'm saying is . . . why do they want people to come up with the money in the beginning?

Mrs. Balasingam added:

> But it's not all . . . it depends on your earning income, right? It depends on how much you're earning, not all parents can top up S$50 a month. So if it's going by the rate of a dollar-per-dollar match, the more you put in . . . of course the more you benefit. But I got other things to worry about day to day. I can't think about how I can keep this money in the bank for future use when day to day is already a problem for me.

Similar observations were made by other respondents. For instance, Mr. and Mrs. Lee, the Chinese couple with a combined monthly household income of more than S$10,000 who reflected on the tax rebates earlier, reflected on the CDA scheme. Mrs. Lee said:

> I think Singapore government is very careful even when they give benefits. Other than the S$3,000 cash, they have another which is top-up, dollar-matching. That is provided . . . you have the money in the account. So not many families can enjoy that, especially the lower income, so at the end of the day the government is careful in a sense that . . . They [the government] are too careful. I mean, they won't want low-income families to have very large, many kids in that sense, so I only see that unless you have the money that you can put it in the bank then you get the additional money from them. You must hit a certain income ceiling in order to enjoy such benefits. They are very careful with their spending, that's about it. So they want to help, but they are very careful who should be the ones having babies, in that sense. Very strange.

Mr. Lee added:

> So you get half measures; basically you end up with something like we said that is good if it's there but it doesn't really . . . It doesn't push you to decide to make babies.

Rahimi, an unmarried 27-year-old Malay respondent with a polytechnic diploma, living in a five-room HDB flat, with a monthly household income of S$3,000–3,999, articulated how "disposable income" mediates the effectiveness of the CDA scheme:

> We have problems in disposable income. It's not a problem of all these subsidies and funds. The problem is disposable income, so if we can't survive with our disposable income then we are screwed. That's the way we see it. We need to increase disposable income; that's what we need, and that's what

> will help. The problem is disposable income. That, I think, that's the main thing. So even if all these funds, [including] Edusave, is so-called frozen. Everything is all frozen, so we can't make use of this money. And we have talked to some families who know of all these funds, but this is so-called future. For future. So what about now? How can we talk about future when we can't survive now?

What Rahimi understood about disposable income and what Mr. Lee characterized as the logic of "half measures" did not escape lower-income respondents; indeed, this logic has greater financial implications for them. For example, Mazlan, who told of his friend not knowing about the policies, said, "What I heard is that, for example, if we save a certain amount, the government will match also the amount. But it's very hard for us to [save]."

It is important to note that the data does not suggest that the CDA matching fund is not encouraging per se; the question is *whom* it is encouraging. Indeed, university students described the CDA dollar-for-dollar match scheme as "a good move as it should make people save," and "a step in the right direction." However, they also observed that the effects may be limited and biased, as articulated by Hui Ling:

> What if the parents already have problems settling all the bills that they need for the children, and they will have little money left to contribute to the dollar-for-dollar scheme, which means that they can't really benefit much from it. And then for the richer, if it's not limited to the lower-income, then the richer can contribute as much as they can, and then the doubling would be a lot more. It's like S$10 and S$100. The S$10 becomes S$20, and the S$100 becomes S$200.

Such observations resonate with the logic of what Brown *et al.* (2003: 22–23) have termed "accumulation versus disaccumulation." "Accumulation" means that "very small economic and social advantages can have large cumulative effects over many generations," while "disaccumulation" refers to the less-understood fact that economic disadvantages can also be compounded over time. On the one hand, children in lower-income households are disadvantaged because their parents' disposable income is small, and this disadvantage translates to the deprivation of their CDAs; on the other hand, children in well-off households benefit not only from their parents' higher disposable income, but also from the state's financial contributions. Thus, the CDA scheme plays a role in intergenerational accumulation and disaccumulation of privilege.

In summary, interviewees point out that parents have to use cash to cover items such as education and medical bills that are immediate day-to-day worries. Such expenditures reduce the amount of savings that can be put into CDAs. Only families who can cover these basic expenses can benefit from the matching fund scheme and still have savings and cash liquidity.

Summary

In this chapter, I suggest that the gap between the stated pronatalist policy goal and the outcome of persistent low fertility is at least partly a function of (a) the larger framework in which pronatalist incentives are understood; (b) the channels through which such policy information is disseminated and learned; and (c) the key forms in which financial benefits are distributed and perceived.

To recap, first, respondents' perceptions of cost of living are found to be inversely related to their responses to policy effectiveness with respect to fertility decisions. Second, respondents with a lower level of education (without a university education) were more likely to be completely unaware of such financial subsidies than their counterparts with a university education. Third, there is a perceived class bias in the implementation of existing financial incentives; the perception of the effectiveness of tax rebates is inversely related to property ownership, while the perception of the effectiveness of the Children Development Account matching fund is inversely related to respondents' monthly household income.

The high and rising cost of living provides a lens through which citizens consider whether government policies encourage them to have an additional child. This finding lends support to the theoretical importance of the concept of "framing" in understanding decision-making behavior. While economic growth in Singapore has been generally positive since 2000 (with the exception of 2001), with 8.8, 6.6, and 7.9 percent growth rates in 2004, 2005, and 2006, the fertility rate has remained constant, around 1.25 per woman of childbearing age. This study suggests that policy effectiveness is at least partly a function of citizens' interpretation of policies in relation to inflation associated with economic growth. Which specific dimensions associated with economic recession would shape citizens' responses is an empirical question, although respondents in this study do mention that job insecurity, not deflation, sets the frame in times of recession.[3]

Interview data also show that there is a lack of awareness of various government policies, including the essentials of the Baby Bonus scheme—a policy with the explicit goal of economic support for having a child, particularly among less-educated women of childbearing age. Responses suggest that there is a need to disseminate detailed information about pronatalist incentives in earlier stages of decision making, prior to childbirth in hospitals. Moreover, it is important to broaden the channels of communication, via, for example, sending mail and posting on notice boards in residential buildings, a communication factor that has not been emphasized in the existing literature. Given that the Singaporean government is keenly aware of the critical importance of disseminating such information, the finding that it has not gotten the pronatalist message across may have broader implications for other countries.

Finally, respondents in this study point to perceived class bias in policy mechanisms. On the one hand, respondents who reside in or own private properties disproportionately constitute those who praise tax rebates as a form of pronatalist financial subsidy. On the other, the poor cannot contribute as much as the rich, so the requirement of matching funds (in contrast to a universal child or family allowance, as instituted in Denmark, Sweden, and Finland) is perceived to increase the capacity of higher-income households to have children. Thus, I suggest that a *de facto* "differential class-specific pronatalism" (Drakakis-Smith and Graham 1996; cf. Palen 1986; Wee 1995) continues to be in effect, although it is neither represented as such in policy statements nor analyzed as such in recent studies on Singaporean fertility policies. Perhaps more importantly, household income inequality increased in the 1990s. By the year 2000, when the Baby Bonus scheme was first introduced, the gap was dramatic:

> the ratio of the average income of households in the top 20 per cent to that of households in the lowest 20 percent rose from 11 in 1990 to 21 in 2000. . . . Households in the top 20 percent accounted for larger shares of the total income—from 48 percent in 1990 to 51 percent in 2000.
>
> (Singapore Department of Statistics 2002)

As for the debate on the effectiveness of different measures of financial subsidy noted earlier, this study lends evidence to the claim that tax rebates are positive but limited in their reach. Cash subsidies, if given generously and over the long term, help to directly address concerns about rising cost of living, and are positively associated with individuals' fertility decisions. Future studies might examine the relative effects of lump-sum payments and income-dependent benefits for individuals in different income categories, or statistically compare total benefits for several types of families in a national representative sample. Last, but not least importantly, this chapter has focused on the role of state financial incentives in individual fertility decisions. For a holistic analysis, one needs to take into consideration other institutional factors (such as provisions in work–family balance) as well as cultural factors (such as gender relations and parent-child relations) in understanding pronatalist population policies and individuals' fertility decisions.

5 Privileging the citizen-worker*

The Singaporean government's pronatalist work–family-balance policies—including, but not limited to, maternity leave, paternity leave, and childcare leave policies—are aimed at providing family time to encourage citizens to have more children. However, citizens, as parents and prospective parents, have a litany of questions regarding this: Who is going to provide care for newborns and children? Do women remain the primary caregivers? What are the responsibilities for men? Do institutions play a role?

With the increase in participation of married women in the paid labor force and cuts in state social service provisions, Hochschild (2003) highlighted the problem of "care deficit" and pointed out that the way care deficit is addressed relates to basic ideas and ideals about care: How is care defined? Who should give it? What constitutes sufficient and quality care? Hochschild further suggested that taken together, answers to these questions make up a "cultural model" that drives political discussion and influences the direction of public policy, and she identified four cultural models:

> 1) The *traditional model* represented by the image of the homemaker mother.
> 2) The *post-modern model* represented by the working mother who "does it all" with no additional help from any quarter and no adaptation to her work schedule. This image often goes along with a tacit lowering of standards of care, as well as making those lower standards seem normal.
> 3) The *cold modern model* represented by impersonal institutional care in year-round ten-hour day-care and old-age homes.
> 4) The *warm modern model* in which institutions provide some care for the young and elderly, while women and men join equally in providing private care, as well.
>
> [Emphasis added] (2003: 214)

* Chapter 5 is a modified version of the author's article, "Re-Producing Citizens: gender, employment, and work–family balance policies in Singapore", *Journal of Workplace Rights*, 14(3): 351–374.

In examining assumptions associated with elements of the institutional-cultural model through the lens of these models, I argue that "cultural models" not only underlie caregiving but also influence childbearing decisions among couples. Moreover, at the macro level, cultural ideas are embedded in population policies of the state. Major findings presented in this chapter suggest that Singapore's pronatalist policies supporting work–family balance are premised on the post-modern working mother model, while perceptions and responses of citizens exhibit a mixture of characteristics of the traditional homemaker model and the warm modern gender-egalitarian model.

Diversity in individual aspirations

To begin with, citizens' responses toward such policies vary consistently according to aspirations for a life centered on paid employment or on family, as well as on how they perceive workplace expectations and the consequences of not meeting such expectations. I identify two groups of women respondents based on their answers to semi-structured interview questionnaires. Interviewees were asked to respond to this questionnaire item:

> If you have a child or would like to have a child, your *ideal* choice is to
> 1) not work before and after having a child/children,
> 2) keep working after having a child/children, or
> 3) quit your job after having a child/children.

Interviewers then probed further for justifications. Two research assistants and I coded answers and identified the following two groups of women respondents:

1) Family-oriented women: both married and unmarried women who voluntarily want to quit their jobs when they have children (but may not be able to realize this ideal because of other considerations), and stay-at-home mothers, women who ideally and in real life do not work after marriage and childbearing; and
2) Career-oriented women: women who, ideally, want to keep working after having children.

In other words, I assess a woman's identity pertaining to family or work primarily in terms of whether she would change her behavior temporarily or permanently after childbirth. Among the 114 survey respondents who were unmarried, 72 were career-oriented women who would, ideally, like to continue working after child-birth, and 34 were family-oriented women who would, ideally, quit after childbirth (8 respondents did not give a clear indication of their preference.) Among the 51 survey respondents who were married, 10 were career-oriented and 38 were family-oriented (3 respondents did not give a clear answer).

As will be further elaborated upon in the following section, citizens' responses to government policies vary consistently according to aspirations for a life centered on paid employment or on family, as well as according to the way in which they perceive workplace expectations and consequences of not meeting such expectations. If responses to pronatalist policies vary according to individuals' own aspirations, the question then becomes, of course, which women are likely to be career oriented and which are likely to be family oriented? Data analysis shows that, within each ethnic group, university-educated women are more career oriented than their less highly educated counterparts. Among women without a university education, Chinese women are more family oriented than Malay and Indian women; among university graduates, Malay women are more family oriented than Chinese and Indian women.

In their answers to the following list of open-ended survey questions, the majority of the women interviewed individually did not make evaluative comments about whether the existing maternity leave policy encouraged them to have an additional child:

1) Was there anything the government did that helped you decide to have a child/children? (For married respondents)
2) If you are deciding whether to have a child, is there anything the government can do that will help you decide? (For the unmarried respondents)
3) As far as you know, has the government done anything to help families in Singapore? If yes, can you please tell me what the Singaporean government has done? If no, what do you think needs to be done by the government to help families?
4) As far as you know, are there any government policies that encourage people to have more children? If yes, can you please tell me what those policies are? Which policies do you think actually work? Among these policies, which one(s) do you think are not working? If no, what needs to be done by the government in terms of policies to encourage people to have more children?

Among the 165 interviewees, 26 made evaluative comments (19 replied that the maternity leave policy was effective, while 7 replied that it was not working). While such small numbers do not allow for any conclusive statement, the pattern is that family-oriented women are more likely than career-oriented women to reply positively; conversely, career-oriented women are more likely than their family-oriented counterparts to reply that the existing maternity leave policy is not working. In the text below, I first draw on the responses from these 26 interviewees.

Differential perceptions of paid maternity leave

Why paid maternity leave is welcomed, especially by family-oriented women

Maternity leave is consistently regarded in a positive way by family-oriented women. Mrs. Khaw (Chinese, age 28, university graduate), the mother of one-year-old Nicholas, was employed as a teacher but has become a full-time homemaker. During the interview, she said:

> I think the extended paid maternity leave definitely encourages mothers to have children because they have ease of mind in knowing that 'I have time to look after my child, and at the same time, I wouldn't lose that financial support.' That is a very important policy.

Similarly, family-oriented Mrs. Pang (Chinese, age 46, secondary school education) thought paid maternity leave "actually works" because mothers "can see to the infant." Family-oriented Mrs. Hamid (Malay, age 24, university graduate) concurred:

> Because, being a teacher, you are entitled to at most three months' maternity leave, and after that you are guaranteed a job. It's not like since you take maternity leave, you'll be dismissed from the company. So that is important, especially for households where it's needed for both to work.

Career-oriented Mrs. Lee (Chinese, age 26, university graduate) explained the importance of maternity leave with guaranteed jobs:

> I am a civil servant, so if you're talking about basic things for me, the two months' maternity leave—or even the third month that they are extending now—helps, because it gives me more time to take care of my newly born child.

In summary, extended paid maternity leave is deemed effective because it allows mothers to spend more time with their newborns without losing income. For career-oriented women, however, the effectiveness of such a policy is contingent on a job guarantee—as is the case with government employees, including teachers and civil servants. As we shall see, however, this does not apply to many women working in the private sector.

Why paid maternity leave is ineffective, particularly for career-oriented women

Some citizens, as parents and prospective parents, said that existing paid maternity leave was not effective. The problems associated with such ineffectiveness are primarily the lack of job guarantees and perceived employer discrimination against women who are likely to take maternity leave. For example, career-oriented Yu Ping (Chinese, age 20, university student) had the following exchange with her interviewer:

INTERVIEWER: Among these policies, which one do you think is not working?
YU PING: Maternity leave.
INTERVIEWER: Why?
YU PING: Because companies don't like pregnant people to get leave. Eventually they will get fired. There's no guarantee [of being retained].

Career-oriented Mrs. Khoo (Chinese, age 30, university graduate) concurred:

> The employers may not like the idea of women or their workers being on leave for three months. OK, it's a fact that a lot of bosses don't like to employ mothers or women because they will have three months of maternity leave and then it will affect their work . . . Even though there is this law, there are still women who are actually victims of employers who want to still dismiss them, even though there's this law.

Indeed, job insecurity is one of the main reasons for differences in attitude toward existing maternity leave policies. While 14 out of 72 family-oriented women mentioned such concerns, the figure was higher—21 out of 82—for career-oriented women. Perhaps even more tellingly, career-oriented women were more likely than their family-oriented counterparts to express a desire for maternity leave with legal protection. For instance, career-oriented Mei Ting (Chinese, age 21, university student) explained:

> Because women are facing problems such as employers not wanting them when they are pregnant, perhaps the government can step in to have a law or regulation that will protect women [who are] married and getting pregnant. Because we have heard of employers and people who are criticizing those who are pregnant and not working.

Career-oriented Hui Fen (Chinese, age 22, university student) reinforced this view, suggesting that job security should be a mandatory (*chiang zhi xing*) provision:

> Actually the government already has [maternity leave] policies, but I don't think a lot of couples are making use of such policies . . . some mothers worry that they would be replaced . . . that's why they just cut their maternity leave short. They went back to work one month after they gave birth. It's not very good . . . There should be mandatory job security. I mean, you [i.e., the government] have to set this law that mothers can go for their full maternity leave for three months. How can you [the government] give them [women] the idea that 'I take three months of maternity leave but I may be sacked or replaced'? [If so] I would go back to work after one month. The only worry is that you might lose your job. Paid maternity leave doesn't secure you in your job. You would still lose your job. What's the point for the government to give you $1,000, $2,000 [in terms of paid maternity leave]? You would be losing the $1,000, S$2,000 [i.e., losing your regular income in the long term when you lose your job.]

The perception of job insecurity related to leave taking is pervasive. Sunthari (Indian, age 30, university graduate) commented that:

> there is a catch there [in the maternity leave provision]. Some companies if they do find out—you read all these letters in the [*Straits Times*] Forum and everything—these mothers get terminated the minute they are found out, you know they are expecting, and then three months, a lot of people say, 'Wow, what am I going [to] do without you for three months?'

Latifa, a 20-year-old university student, shared the same sentiment: "Maternity leave . . . [should come with] the certainty that they won't see that as a liability, like they won't discourage you getting promoted or [be instrumental in your] losing your job."

Raziya (Malay, age 20, university student) put it in a positive way: "Women who have careers should have rights. They should be able to take the nine months off and still return to their jobs and be guaranteed that [the jobs are] still there."

In short, more days of maternity leave are particularly welcomed by family-oriented women who ideally would like to quit their jobs and care for their children—but in reality, may not. In contrast, women who ideally want to keep working after having children have strong reservations about existing paid maternity leave, as their concern is the lack of legal protection for their jobs if they take leave. In other words, it is critical to have state protection against dismissal by employers on the grounds of family leave of absence.

Kinds of institutional support sought by women

Family-oriented women were also more likely to suggest flexible work hours and homemaker allowances as additional policy initiatives that would encourage women to consider more births. For instance, Mrs. Kuek (Chinese, age 30, university graduate, monthly household income S$10,000 and above), who has two children but has continued to work, said:

> You need supportive bosses, because if you have children, it also means that sometimes you need to go back [home] early. There's a need to strike a better balance in work. I wouldn't be able to stay in the office for 12 hours a day.

Kadijah (Malay, age 21, university student) said:

> What the government can do for me is in terms of my working time . . . There should be flexibility in my working time. Help me be there for my children . . . and at the same time still contribute to the economy.

Mrs. Hamid (Malay, age 24, university graduate), a contract teacher with one child, sees flexible working hours and on-site childcare centers as options:

> Flexible working hours that I can clock in anytime, any day, or even the ability to work from home. Or, even if I can't work from home, maybe a childcare center at the workplace [would encourage me to have another child] . . . so

> instead of sending my child somewhere else and go to work, I can just bring them.

Interview data also suggest that the culture of long work hours underlies respondents' requests to have institutionalized flexible work hours. Average work hours are longer in the sales and service sector than in the manufacturing sector. At the same time, as we saw in Chapter 3, the sales and service sector is the sector in which numbers of jobs have grown and will grow. Rashida (Malay, age 21, university student), who, ideally, wants to keep working after having children, articulates how the reality of long hours undermines the rhetoric of work–life balance:

> Government incentives . . . OK, they have been going on and on with the work-life balance thing, but by the look of it, it's not exactly true. You are still expected to work beyond the working hours even during weekdays. From what I notice, when I go to these recruitment talks, you have to work like [up to] 8 [pm], sometimes you have to work 24–7. I mean, the government says that it is a five-day week and weekends you can be with the family and stuff. But you have to be realistic here.

Similarly, Meena (Indian, age 34, university graduate) suggested that "They [the government] would really need to look into the number of hours, especially I feel for mothers; they really have to be mindful that the mothers really don't take home any work to do." She added:

> The government has this thing called 'Eat with your Family Day,' which I personally feel is so ridiculous because you promote that one day in the entire year, out of 365 days, to eat with your family—so everybody has to go home, your employers are not supposed to keep you in school or at work, or wherever, and then you are supposed to go eat with your family for one day; then what happens to the rest of the time?

In other words, these respondents articulated the need for the "right to request flexi-work" that is available in the British Employment Act or the "right to shorter and flexible working hours" included in the Norwegian Working Environment Act.

Finally, respondents suggested that the government provide allowances for stay-at-home mothers, which is in line with the idea of "care allowances" mentioned in Chapter 1. Indeed, as can be seen from the following interview data, respondents tended to be aware of the practice of state-provided homemaker allowances in other countries. Mrs. Yap (Chinese, age 41, upper secondary), who has two children, articulated:

> There seems to be no relief for homemakers. It's a bit tough for just one person to bring in the bread and butter. But again, you know, to give the best quality time and everything to your children. So I think probably the government

> should look into this, not just giving incentives to those parents who return to work. I mean, comparatively to my sister-in-law in Australia. She's stay-home, and she has like a monthly 300 Aussie dollars, they call it 'nappy money' or whatever, you know! [Laughs] Stay-home mother they have that kind of incentives, so it's very good!

Mrs. Osman (Malay, age 33, polytechnic diploma) added:

> It's good if they can give housewife some allowance. Even [if] it means S$100 or S$150 per month . . . it's still an allowance for housewife. 'Cos doesn't mean housewife we don't contribute anything to the society, we do, that's why we bring up our own kids to make sure that do something for the society . . . The best is for the parents to bring up their kids and you know, as a housewife, we are also contributing by bringing up the next generation. At least as a housewife, you feel that you are being appreciated in bringing up the future generation. And in fact . . . European countries are actually doing that.

The interviewees put forth several reasons to underscore the need for a homemaker allowance. First, even though "it's a bit tough for just one person to bring in the bread and butter," women choose to stay at home to "give the best quality time and everything to your children," sometimes at the expense of their own careers. Second, a homemaker allowance serves as an official recognition that stay-at-home mothers also contribute to society. Third, expenses for children's education continue despite a lack of mothers' income; state subsidies would help to defray some of these costs.

Varying responses toward paid paternity leave

Paid paternity leave is not crucial for most men

Extra days of paternity leave would help, but this is not the deciding factor for fathers and prospective fathers when they are considering an additional child. Men place more emphasis on financial concerns than paternity leave days. This is reflected in the focus group discussions. For instance, Mr. Lee (Chinese, age 36, university graduate, S$10,000 and above) said:

> Giving parents leave and all that, it's definitely good, but then again, it's not something that will push the couple to have kids. Having kids is a long-term [commitment], it's not [as if] three days leave [from work] will tilt the balance to make you decide to have more kids.

The way that child rearing is perceived by men is primarily predicated on the role of fathers as breadwinners, as Mr. Balasingam (Indian, age 34, other diploma, S$4,000–4,999) articulated:

> The fact of life is, when you're married, [the] father is supposed to provide bread and butter, so everything is money. Although some people may think it's not so, but that's the reality of life. If you cannot provide for the family, you're a failure. Your wife will ask you: 'Why [do] you want kids? Why should we have more kids when you will not be able to fulfill the [financial responsibility]?' If I can't convince my wife . . . [when] women become mothers, they are very concerned about their children and not their husbands. They want to know whether their child will have adequate medical [care], if you can't do something, as a husband . . . you're going to get hell when you go back [return home].

The pressure of the provider role is keenly felt by some men. Mr. Khaw (Chinese, age 30, university graduate, S$4,000–4,999) and Mrs. Khaw describe how the longer working hours of the father—in Mr. Khaw's case, as a teacher—when the children were still young led to a misunderstanding between them:

MR. KHAW: Right now, even government [work is] based on performance. So you increase your performance, you get your performance bonus. And it's all these performance bonuses that come in now to help me cover [her no-pay] leave . . . So it makes me work harder, which means I've less time to spend [with my family], and she knows it, she feels it. Morning, 6-something, I'm off. I come back 7, 8pm sometimes. So for us, as much as I would like to be with the family, I know I also have to be in school because if my performance is seen as good, I get a bonus and that bonus can help me out later on. So these are the things that stress us because . . . she'll complain, and I'll say "You don't understand what I'm trying to do."

MRS. KHAW: So I always tell him, "Oh, so this is all you say to him [their son, Nicholas]—'Hi!' 'Bye!' 'Good night'!" So you know, the interaction, the hushing him to sleep, changing the diapers . . . all these [are the responsibilities of] the mother. I mean, I feel that sometimes, as a child it would be nice to know that my daddy was part of bringing me up.

In the private sector, a focus group interview with university students—Thomas (Chinese, age 22, S$10,000 and above) and Chuan Hock (Chinese, age 25, S$4,000–4,999)—highlights the predominant views of work demands in the private sector in Singapore. Thomas wanted to have two children, but he warned that he would not take leave from work, so as "not to influence my position in my job." Indeed, even if more leave days are were provided for in government policy, he said "it all depends on the bosses . . . Your boss says 'I want you back tomorrow,' you've got to be back tomorrow no matter what the government says."

Chuan Hock, too, was skeptical about the prospects for a more generous leave policy:

> You're in Singapore. In Singapore, you need to work, you don't work you die . . . Even if the government gives support, cool. What about the private sector? How are they going to react to it?

This skepticism was echoed in the focus group discussion, quoted below, with university students Chee Keong (Chinese, age 24, university graduate, S$8,000–8,999) and his girlfriend, Hui Lin (age 22), who were both anticipating a demanding life in the corporate world, especially in light of their own aspirations. Chee Keong said:

> I think it's very hard for the government to help in terms of the labor market, because it's really your personal wants and what you really want to achieve. Say I'm going to work as an auditor. My job is from 9 to 5, but because I want to go up the corporate ladder, I will work harder. Even if there's this thing called the five-day week, how many people really work five days, other than civil servants? So it's really about our personal wants. It's not so much what the government can [do to] help. They can give us guys maternity [*sic*] leave, but will I go for maternity [*sic*] leave? I will not go, right?

Hui Lin also highlighted the role of work pressures:

> Especially in Singapore, where everything is so work-based, it's efficiency-based. So it's very hard to [take] leave. You're worried about your work, and you're worried about your kid. It's very stressful. The whole environment in Singapore is very stressful, actually.

For his part, Chee Keong also expects little empathy from male corporate leaders:

> How many married men really take care of the kids? Seriously, let's say the CEO of any company. How much time does he have to take care of the kids when you're seeing the CEO there every day? I mean, for a corporate world, for a private company, would the CEO want to encourage family life more, or does he want to encourage the employee to work harder? I'm sure the CEO wants to encourage the employee to work harder. So that would be at the top of his mind, even if he's a married man.

Thus, there is a palpable sense that men feel they are primarily responsible for being breadwinners; for better-educated and higher-income men, these pressures are exacerbated by their own job expectations. The responsibility of being breadwinners, however, seems even more difficult for men in the lower-income households to meet because of a lack of job security. For example, Mr. Chong (Chinese, age 49, no formal education, S$2,000–2,999) made the following observation with regard to young couples' unwillingness to have an additional child:

> It was because the economic environment was not as bad as it is now. It was very easy to find a job then. Firstly, there was no problem in finding odd jobs and so on. Now, when you are asking for an odd job, people would first ask how old you are and carried on by saying, 'No, we hire Chinese [i.e., new labor immigrants from the People's Republic of China] here.' The Chinese provide

> very cheap labor. They would tell me that they can hire three Chinese workers with S$30 but only one worker with the same amount if they were to hire me. So one should not think of the issue of children if he cannot even find an odd job.

Similarly, Mr. Idris (Malay, age 40, secondary high school, S$3,000–3,999), Mrs. Ibrahim (Malay, age 49, upper secondary high school, S$2,000–2,999), and Mr. Ibrahim (Malay, age 52, secondary high school, S$3,000–3,999) attributed the reluctance of couples to consider an additional child to retrenchment, which they saw as potentially detrimental to child rearing. Following is an excerpt from the interview:

MR. IDRIS: Job-wise, is it going to be a sure thing that we still got a job, whatever, you know.

MRS. IBRAHIM: Nowadays retrench here and there, we won't know, you see. Not like last time, we can stay at one place. But now . . .

MR. IBRAHIM: Problem is the work. Work very uncertain . . . Work very unstable nowadays. Anytime, any day, you can get retrenched, right? That's the problem. Once you [are] retrenched, how are you going to bring up the children? School them? You can see yourself. In Singapore, I think nowadays half of the workforce is foreigners.

In short, job insecurity is also seen as a problem by men in middle-income households, and there seems to be a perception that there is a generational difference in the job market for Singaporeans.

Why paternity leave is sought by some men as a national program

While male respondents clearly view the financial burden of childbearing and child rearing as a central concern, they also think there are good reasons—such as supporting their wives—for paternity leave to be extended.

Moreover, as the following excerpt shows, the best practices of other countries are emphasized. Mr. Khaw advocates longer paid paternity leave to take into consideration medical uncertainty in births:

MRS. KHAW: I think it's interesting how Singapore only gives three months of paid leave to women. It shows a bit about how our society looks at the roles of woman as a main caregiver . . . [.] The parents are telling me that in China, both, I think both the mum and the dad get a total of eight months' paid leave. And it's transferable. So it goes to show that the government looks at the family unit as both the father and mother are equally responsible in bringing up a child. And I think it works both ways. If the government were to support that, then the father will start to take up more caregiving responsibilities. But if the policy is such that we only give women paid leave, then the man has to work harder. I've to work with what the policy . . . with what is given to us.

MR. KHAW: Only two days and three days of paternity leave is quite pathetic. It creates that thing like OK, the man don't [*sic*] need to worry, the mother will look after. But the mother needs to recover.

MODERATOR: So, if the government increases paid leave days, will that help you cope with family?

MR. KHAW: Definitely. It's more being able to be with your family and the newborn at that period of time. I think the initial stage can be very important. I thank God that there are no complications, but if there were complications at that point of time, then three days, then after that is taking leave from work and may not even be paid for it.

In a similar vein, Mr. Balasingam and Mrs. Balasingam (Indian, age 34, upper secondary, S$4,000–4,999) talked about family "bonding." An excerpt from the interview illustrates this:

MR. BALASINGAM: Obviously to bond with the family. To change diapers, help the mum, so as to lessen postnatal stress for her. When the child is born, we can spend time together. At least we know that there is some bonding and we can talk . . .

MRS. BALASINGAM: Yah, the mother is very stressed . . .

MR. BALASINGAM: Stressed after she gives birth.

MRS. BALASINGAM: A new mother, right? First child I go through the trauma alone, second child I go again alone, third child . . . how long you want me to continue going alone?

Among young unmarried male respondents, Yong Hai (Chinese, age 25, university graduate) was in favor of longer paid paternity leave "to spend time with your kids and wife. Because during the time, she will need a lot of moral support from the husband." Kalimuthu (Indian, age 22, university student) emphasized, "I feel that [paternity leave is] not really for the child per se but it's to support my wife. In that sense, paternity leave would be important because [without it] you are making your wife go through it all alone." Naser (Indian, age 23, university student) had the same opinion:

> I would have to agree. Maybe not like three-month paternity leave, but . . . a week or so would be realistic. I mean, in this day and age where almost everyone is focused on efficiency and productivity, no one is going to give three months' paternity leave.

For some respondents, becoming a father means actual involvement with their wives and children in addition to being good providers for the family. For instance, when the interviewer asked Seng Wah (Chinese, age 24, other diploma) whether he would feel disconnected to the workplace if he took paternity leave, he replied:

> Depends from company to company. Let's say if your company has a good team or as in working with a team and the team can cover up your job for that . . . of course I'm not looking at months in replacement for three days. I'm talking like maybe one week.

Thus, these male respondents would be encouraged by a slightly longer paternity leave, with a week as the most frequently mentioned figure.

Doubts about paternity leave can be further allayed if such leave is legislated and treated similarly to the National Service "in-camp training" policy—that is, applied across the board rather than left to the company's discretion. In Singapore, not only do male citizens undergo two years' compulsory full-time military service when they reach the age of 18, but they are also required to report annually for up to 40 days a year for in-camp reservist training to the age of 50 for commissioned officers, and 40 for others. All public organizations and private-sector companies must allow National Service men to fulfill their reservist duties without taking unpaid leave; the government pays their salaries for the duration of their training period.

As Ismail (Malay, age 24, polytechnic diploma) explained:

> Even though I work in a private sector, I got the paternity leave. I think it's helpful [in encouraging people to have more children]. It's the same like for a guy who work in a private sector has to go for the reservist. It's the same. If this is a government policy I shouldn't be worried [about taking leave]. If the government manages to implement this policy like the reservist policy, this shouldn't be a problem because it can be like a standard thing in every company whether it is a private or public sector, if the government can successfully implement this policy.

Notably, the idea of implementing one week's paid paternity leave in a manner akin to reservist training is repeatedly suggested. In other words, men are in favor of state legislation to take away company discretion that may not support the taking of paternity leave. Mr. Owyong, a 55-year-old Singaporean–Chinese company owner with a teenage daughter, summed up the necessity for a state legislative provision:

> Manpower, they [companies] try to stretch each individual to prolong their working hour. They don't mind paying a little bit more, because that is a controllable [amount] . . . except those like the NS [National Service] men. They [companies] have no other alternative; there's a law, by law that the employee has to go.

Thus, a number of interviewees—fathers and prospective fathers—do appreciate the demands that come with fatherhood; they also look for more institutional support from both the state and private sector.

Women's and men's perceptions of childcare leave

In this section, I present interview data on the effectiveness of pronatalist childcare leave incentives. Three themes have emerged repeatedly from the findings: First, in terms of provision, the current childcare leave policy is seen as insufficient and should be extended to include school-age children, rather than restricted to children under seven years of age. Second, incentives should be provided to mothers and fathers separately as their individual entitlements. Third, in terms of financing days of leave, respondents suggest that the government should pay.

Mr. and Mrs. Ravindran had the following lively exchange in which Mrs. Ravindran shared her experience as a human resource manager having to answer questions from her colleague regarding restrictive childcare leave:

MRS. RAVINDRAN: I also think they [the government] are giving paid childcare leave for children below seven. That is not good enough! What about children who are eight years and nine years and ten years and eleven years? They will fall sick, you know. You think they don't fall sick?

MR. RAVINDRAN: But you know, practically, we have to have a cut-off mark.

MRS. RAVINDRAN: No, I think as long as the child is school-going, you [the government] must give. So if my son is Secondary 1 and he's sick, I don't have to take leave to look after him? Of course you have to! The other day I had to rush to school to bring him back because he was vomiting in school. So that's why I say the below seven thing doesn't make sense. Are you trying to say older kids don't get sick? It's not encouraging at all! Are you telling me that your son in Primary 2, 3, 4 don't fall sick? We take our own leave!

So when you give something, you give fully . . . They [the government] just cannot give something and hold back other thing, no. You give, give for everyone. I'm not saying give for university or give for junior college. I'm just saying let the cut-off be secondary school. One of the staff [in my company] asked me, "So are you telling me my child won't fall sick?" I said "No, this is the government rule, not my rule."

I really think they give some leeway, they [the government] make it like they're so stingy with it. And the thing is people are not happy! They ask, "Are you saying my son is not a child anymore at ten years old?"

At this point in the exchange, Mr. Ravindran raised an interesting question that was also brought up in other interviews: "Maybe they [the government] are afraid of abuse?" Mrs. Ravindran replied, "Take it from me, when you have kids you don't abuse the system." But Mr. Ravindran was not ready to defer yet: "Hang on, you never know. There are parents who use that as an excuse to gallivant." This remark goaded Mrs. Ravindran into giving the following reply:

> If that's the case, [the government] should not give even two days. How do you know a mother with four-year-old child is not abusing the childcare leave? You don't know that. So you cannot suspect and say only seven-year-old and

below can take leave. If your fourteen-year-old child got dengue fever, does that mean you don't have to go care for your child?

Mr. Ravindran then said, "They [the government] should address it [the restriction on childcare leave days to children aged below seven]." The notion that the provision of childcare leave should be extended is echoed in other interviews, although suggestions vary. Some advocated extending such leave to children in primary school, while others recommended that it should be extended to children in secondary school.

Moreover, it would be helpful if mothers and fathers were individually entitled to a certain number of childcare leave days, as kindergarten teacher Mrs. Visvanathan (Indian, age 48, S$1,000–1,999) explained in the following focus group discussion, together with Mr. Nair (Indian, age 59, other diploma, S$5,000–5,999) and Mrs. Nair (Indian, age 51, university graduate):

MR. NAIR: When they [the children] were small? When the one year, five years, two or three [childcare leave] days [a year] is enough. Because why you know, because my wife is not working.

ALL: Ah, yes.

MODERATOR: But for working parents, from your experience?

MR. NAIR: Working parents is a different case.

MODERATOR: What do you think?

MRS. VISVANATHAN: Definitely, you see, at least five days. Individual, individual [entitlement]. Because I have seen, they [parents] will come with leave . . . then I will see, today, oh your daddy is taking leave. Even the little children can tell, oh today my mummy is looking after me. So at least five days for the father and five days for mother. At the age, from the beginning, at least eighteen months, we [the kindergartens] start from eighteen months to five years, child will fall sick like anything.

Similarly, in the focus group discussion with Mr. and Mrs. Khaw, Mr. Khaw made the point that small children were particularly prone to fall sick when placed in childcare centers, and suggested that leave policies should encourage both parents to take care of children. Mr. Khaw said:

> I think children's illnesses can come and go. We don't know. When you put in infant care . . . within a month, three or four times, because after the first week maybe he still hasn't recovered and you go again. We need to stagger. Maybe the husband goes once, the wife goes once. You cannot always ask the wife to take the leave.

This point echoed the concern that women have with leave-taking. As Hui Fen said:

> The government must let the company know that the worker cannot be replaced. Then the worker can have a standing [secured status] in the company.

> If you work all the way up . . . are you willing to give your job up? If you give birth you may lose your job. Seriously . . . those with family . . . the boss does not take you seriously . . . I mean for women. Because women tend to care for the family more than men . . . so anything is the mother go [so if anything happens, it's the mother who needs to take time off from the workplace to attend to the child]. It's not the father. Have you ever seen [the] father go? If the school calls, [it] is the mother who leaves work. Mothers take leave, take urgent leave . . . Then, the boss doesn't like it. The mother has to be on time to pick up the child, to leave the workplace, so the boss doesn't like it. If one has to rush home to cook, the boss doesn't like it. Even though the boss may have children, it's different when it comes to his employees.

Finally, it is important that childcare leave days be paid for by the government rather than financed by employers. As Mrs. Balasingam (age 34, diploma holder) said:

> I'm working longer hours, but I think this is the time [when the child is sick] that I need to spend time with my kid. They need me, but I'm not able to be there as I need to go to work. Even if he falls [really] sick, I take no-pay leave . . . no-pay leave, no-pay leave, then who's going to have the pay?

The question becomes that of how to finance such leave. Mrs. Ravindran articulated the need to extend such leave provision: "The government must come with the fund because if you just ask companies to do this, they will never do this."

Mrs. Ravindran's idea that private enterprises will not provide childcare leave if there is no government support reveals a significant obstacle in helping individuals balance work and family responsibilities. In what follows, I highlight a dialogue in a focus group interview with a young Chinese couple, Mr. Wong and Mrs. Wong (Chinese, both age 27, university graduates, S$6,000–6,999), illustrating dilemmas faced by employers, especially owners of small and medium-sized enterprises.

MRS. WONG: For my organization [a multinational company], we actually have five [days] per child. But it's childcare sick leave. It's only when the child is sick that you are entitled to the sick leave. You know, from my colleagues' perspective, from those who have children, they wouldn't want to take MC [Medical-Certificate warranted leave], because they are afraid that they would be penalized. I guess the employer wouldn't explicitly punish you in a way. But perhaps at the end of the year, they might take into consideration that you are on too many days of MC.

MR. WONG: But in an employer's view, it's quite disturbing when the child is sick, and they take leave, and there's no one to cover her job.

MRS. WONG: This is the problem of Singapore culture . . . Singapore's employment culture. As compared to the other countries, as in maybe London. I have a friend. She's working in London, and she mentioned that her colleague, who's actually a Singaporean, actually wants to quit her Singapore job and she wants to settle in London, because the employers there are very pro-family. It's like [in the case of] her pregnancy; they actually have a room for her to rest. Because pregnancy stage is actually very tiring, so they will actually allow her to nap for one or two hours and things like that. And London's maternity [leave] is like six months or whatever, so I guess the employer is very nice in a way whereby you can actually go off when you finish your work, just to spend time with your family. You don't need to stay until 5:30 when it's the official time to knock off.

MR. WONG: You cannot compare Western country and Asian country.

MRS. WONG: You see, this is the mentality of a Chinese employer, I mean, Singapore's employer.

MR. WONG: We [the employers] are the ones who suffer. For small companies, small organization, we are the ones suffering.

MRS. WONG: Because they are very lean. They only have two or three support staff, so that's why when one is down, then . . .

MR. WONG: That's why the boss has to know all the things.

MRS. WONG: So that he can take over. I guess in a way, like the childcare sick leave, it can be something like the last four weeks of the maternity [leave] whereby the government pay for it, in order to help the SME [small and median-sized enterprises]. Because to the employer, it's a loss to them, so we can actually compensate.

A number of important themes are reflected in the little "argument" between Mrs. Wong and her husband. Mrs. Wong criticizes what she sees as the unsympathetic view of employers toward employees taking childcare sick leave, blaming it on "Singapore culture" or the "employment culture" in Singapore, especially when compared with practices elsewhere. However, Mr. Wong, himself an employer, attempts to elaborate on the difficulties faced by the company whose work responsibilities cannot be adequately covered. The point that both of them make, however, is that a proper or adequate system of childcare sick leave cannot be instituted without government support.

Summary

I suggest that the thrust of state policies and the needs of parents and prospective parents are at variance with each other. To illustrate this divergence, I shall expand the discussion using Hochschild's framework. On one hand, the post-modern supermom model underlies work–life-balance policy initiatives in Singapore. Interviewees point out that there are more benefits for working mothers compared to stay-at-home mothers. In addition, there is no provision for paternity leave (except three days for civil servants), and interviewees observe that active involvement on the part of the father is generally discouraged. These responses suggest that the state adopts a post-modern "supermom" model—a model in which working mothers receive little help in childcare from their spouses. At the same time, the principal assumptions of state policies do not sit well with those who face real dilemmas of meeting demands from both work and family; their responses echo elements of Hochschild's warm modern gender-egalitarian model, in which "institutions provide some care of the young and elderly, while women and men join equally in providing private care, as well."

Moreover, as Hakim (2003) points out, a critical step is to inquire into and acknowledge the emerging diversity of individual orientations toward family and paid employment. This chapter finds that some women would, ideally, like to quit their jobs when they have children, and some would, ideally, not want to quit their jobs. Likewise, while most men still treat their financial responsibility to the family as primary, some articulate the importance of spending time with their families as well. Work–life-balance policies are most effective in meeting the needs of family-oriented women, but not career-oriented women, stay-at-home mothers, or men; in other words, these groups are not encouraged by state initiatives to have more children.

Family-oriented women are more likely than their career-oriented counterparts to suggest that paid maternity leave encourages mothers to have more children, largely because it allows mothers to spend time with their newborns without losing their income. However, the provision of paid maternity leave is insufficient to encourage career-oriented women, who, ideally, want to keep working after having children. For example, they perceive taking paid maternity leave as jeopardizing job security or promotion. Career-oriented women do not lack a sense of family attachment, but do place significant importance on their paid employment. Without a guarantee of job security, they view the work–life-balance policies as inadequate.

In addition, responses from working women indicate that they are aware of—and do not shy away from—the demands of both work and family. However, they need help from the state to make it possible for them to meet such demands successfully; specifically, respondents propose institutional provision of on-site childcare centers so that working mothers can easily visit their children, and flexible work hours so that parents can attend to their children if care is required at home.

With respect to joint efforts of men and women in providing familial private care, while men with stay-at-home wives do not find the lack of paternity leave unsatisfactory, other men articulate the ideal and reality of involved fatherhood, and suggest that longer paid paternity leave and more routine family time would be helpful. Moreover, they suggest specific ways in which paid paternity leave provision can be effective. By frequently invoking the analogy of the National Service reservist policy, they are implicitly asking the state to treat childbearing and child rearing as a top national priority.

Understanding how individuals in different groups respond to policies becomes even more important if we take into account the following statistics. In 2005, of all married couples in Singapore, 44 percent were dual-career couples; 36 percent were husband/breadwinner–wife/homemaker couples; 5.5 percent had wives as sole breadwinners; and 14.5 percent had no income earners (Ministry of Community Development, Youth, and Sports 2008).

Finally, it is important that leave provisions be financed by the government rather than paid for by employers; this is one of the key ways in which the state can support individuals in ensuring that their paid employment will, at a minimum, not be jeopardized by childbearing and the responsibilities of child rearing.

The fact that, in this study, only women— not men—articulated the need for structural accommodations in the workplace may reflect the fact that, in Singapore, gender role relations in the family remain traditional. State policies, however, can either maintain the status quo or channel behaviors in new directions. Given that citizens are suggesting specific ways to encourage a more egalitarian sharing of roles, such as longer paid paternity leave and individual entitlement to childcare leave days, the law's function of disciplining corporate behaviors in this instance is welcomed, so that fathers, should they wish, can be enabled to care for their children.

6 Constructing children's multi-dimensional qualities

> Do we have the time? Do we have the financial resources? Will we be able to save in the future? I think these are the concerns that we have before we consider having a child. But it's also because we don't want to have only one child . . .
>
> Mr. Khaw (age 30, Chinese, university graduate), the father of one-year-old Nicholas

Quantity–quality of children

In this chapter, I examine how socio-cultural constructions of desired "qualities" of children figure in the decision-making process. Becker (1960) first introduced the idea that affluent families seem to substitute quality for quantity in spending more income on each child's rearing and education. This analysis was later expanded by Becker and Lewis (1973) and Becker and Tomes (1976). A key proposition of the quantity–quality of children fertility model is an interaction between quantity and quality such that budget constraints lead to rising marginal costs of quality and engender a trade-off between quality and quantity. The idea of a "quantity–quality trade-off" subsequently generated an extensive body of literature examining the mechanisms that facilitate the trade-off (Alwin 1991; Black 1981, 1989; Retherford and Sewell 1991; Steelman 1985; Zajonc and Markus 1975), was used to account for macro-level phenomena such as poverty (Galor and Moav 2002; Moav 2001), and spawned a sustained debate on whether the trade-off is a causal or spurious relationship (Downey 1995; Guo and VanWey 1999).

Upon closer examination, however, the "quality" aspect of the theory tends to be overwhelmingly measured in terms of children's educational attainment (Downey 1995; Ahlburg, Kelley, and Mason 1996), and, to some extent, their projected income and wealth (Black, Devereux, and Salvanes 2005). For instance, in Blake's influential 1981 study, child quality is measured solely in terms of educational outcomes. More recently, De Tray (2001: S81) noted that:

> constructing an operational measure of child quality is a more difficult task. One approximate measure . . . is the expected full wealth of the child. The

> best available statistic summarizing a child's future economic prospects is the amount of education that child will receive.

The equation of children's "quality" primarily with "human capital" formation (Becker 1964) and financial ability is not without its critics. For instance, Coleman (1988) argues for a deeper understanding of the importance of social capital in the creation of human capital:

> Just as physical capital is created by changes in materials to form tools that facilitate production, human capital is created by changes in persons that bring about skills and capabilities that make them able to act in new ways . . . Social capital, however, comes about through changes in relations among persons that facilitate action. If physical capital is wholly tangible, being embodied in observable material form, and human capital is less tangible, being embodied in the skills and knowledge acquired by an individual, social capital is less tangible yet, for it exists in the relations among persons. Just as physical capital and human capital facilitate productive activity, social capital does as well. For example, a group within which there is extensive trustworthiness and extensive trust is able to accomplish much more than a comparable group without that trustworthiness and trust.

In addition, as Jones (2004: 2) pointed out in his argument for more equal access to education:

> There is currently a ferment of competing concepts of human well-being and disadvantage. Led by development economists such as Amartya Sen and Richard Jolly, the United Nations Development Programme (UNDP) promoted its Human Development Index in order to broaden the traditional emphasis on income.

Thorne (1999) suggested that the overarching concern with human capital is a consequence of major transformations in the global economy which entail an intensification of children's lives:

> . . . in an age-segmented twist of the commodification of everything . . . markets in child products and services are now flourishing in metropolitan areas like Oakland, with an array of private schools, preschools, daycare centers, camps, lessons, housekeepers, nannies, au pairs, paid domestic workers, household "organizers" (who will tidy up closets and drawers), birthday party planners, and taxi and van companies willing to move kids across long distances. In short, a privatized infrastructure for raising children has consolidated, with access and quality depending on one's ability to pay.

In a parallel fashion, "motherhood" has also intensified (Hays 1996). In Singapore, Straughan (2008: 70) suggested that "expectations of motherhood have intensified in our child-centric society, where capitalism continues to propagate the ideology of the sacred child." Lareau (2002: 747) provided ethnographic data collected in the United States to illustrate how practices of parenthood and experiences of childhood vary by class:

> Middle-class parents engage in concerted cultivation by attempting to foster children's talents through organized leisure activities and extensive reasoning. Working-class and poor parents engage in the accomplishment of natural growth, providing the conditions under which children can grow but leaving leisure activities to children themselves.

More recent studies have continued to document the experiences of "intensive mothering" and childhood in middle- and upper-middle class neighborhoods in North America (Blackford 2004; Caputo 2007; Chin 2000). This chapter explores dynamics between childrearing concerns (including but not limited to children's educational attainment) and childbearing decisions. Citizens' own interpretation and understanding of parenthood and "quality of children," in turn, helps to shed light on the larger question of interconnections between state pronatalist policies and their effects on individual fertility behavior.

Interpersonal competence and individual competitiveness

Interview data from 165 women indicate that two considerations figure in respondents' childbearing reasoning. On the one hand, there is a concern with raising a child to excel in an increasingly competitive world. On the other hand, there is a concern that a child should be able to relate to, and cooperate with others, in order to better develop moral character and good citizenship—and this is often given as a reason for having a number of children. Among the 165 interviewees, 13 articulate the former idea, which might be called "individual competitiveness," while 16 articulate the latter idea of "interpersonal competence." In the focus group discussions, these two different conceptualizations of desirable traits in children have even more salient presence. In what follows, I summarize these ideals of "interpersonal competence" and "individual competitiveness" along two dimensions: what it means for the parent as well as for the child.

Companionship and interpersonal competence

One of the most consistent reasons for respondents, as parents and prospective parents, to have or desire to have more than one child is that "one is so lonely."[1] For example, Mr. and Mrs. Khaw already have a boy and they made a conscious decision to have a second child. They made it a point to say that this is *not* because of the pronatalist incentives. As Mr. Khaw says:

> Do we have the time? Do we have the financial resources? Will we be able to save in the future? I think these are the concerns that we have before we

> consider having a child. But it's also because we don't want to have only one child and then the child is the only person with no brother or sister as a support. So I think at least for the both of us we agree that we'll have at least two kids. At the very least.

Mrs. Khaw lamented "Just look at our parents' time. They have like four, five, six siblings and it's such a warm family. And we were thinking, poor Nicholas."

Beyond just keeping the first child company, married respondents in the focus group interviews mentioned practical considerations that an additional sibling could provide, for example, the child would have a confidante. As Mrs. Fong (age 48, Chinese, S$3,000–3,999) with three children, explained that:

> as the time goes by, you watch the elder one grow. I felt that she was getting lonely and then she learned to talk, she started to talk to toys. You can feel that she was lonely. So we said, why not we have another one. It will be much better to have some companion at home to share. You know there are just some things you cannot tell with your parents.

The child might also have an additional source of financial assistance. When asked by the moderator "What is the difference between friends and siblings? . . . you can even borrow from your friends," Mrs. Govindan (age 59, Indian, S$1,000–1,999/month) replied, "you can ask your friends for money, yes, they'll give you. Your family members, you tell them your problem, they'll give you the money if they have the money. You don't have to ask." In a similar vein, Mr. Idris (age 40, Malay, S$3,000–3,999/month) gave a personal example to explain why he wanted more than one child: "I've got four brothers, so any problem, we have each other. You know, when you need somebody to help you, financial or whatever, my brothers are there for me." Finally, an additional child helps to secure the family line, as Mr. Wong (age 27, Chinese, S$6,000–6,999/month) remarked, "I think one boy is not enough for family, because boys go for the National Service. There's some danger involved. One boy is not enough, I think, to carry on the family line. Must be two boys."

Unmarried respondents also bring up the issue of "one is too lonely,"[2] but not practical implications. Instead, they articulate their belief that having an additional child would help children develop qualities related to "interpersonal competence." In a focus group discussion, Nadra and Siti Isah, two 22-year-old Malay female university students, gave examples to elaborate on how having several siblings is not just a matter of creating a warmer environment at home, but also fostering a child's moral character and intellectual development.

NADRA: I think there're some things a child can learn having another sibling around. It helps in their development. It's different from when they're own their own.

MODERATOR: Can you give some examples?

NADRA: Taking care of one another, looking after each other's needs, not just thinking about yourself, which is kind of what I picked out along the way.

MODERATOR: And what about you? Do you have a reason why it has to be two or three [children]?

SITI ISAH: Many reasons. I've seen many single children, my friends who don't have siblings and they usually complain of being too lonely, not having anyone at home. Then there's a risk of over-pampering your child if there's only one child. And like what she said, there're some things the child can learn from having siblings. Learning how to compromise, living with other people, give and take, learn to share and besides the social development of the child, it's also for intellectual development. Having siblings help the child to develop all this.

MODERATOR: What's the difference between having siblings and having friends?

SITI ISAH: It's more obvious when you're young. When you grow up and you're out in school and you can go out with your friends, there's a different kind. But when you're young, you can't go out on your own, so the only development you have is within the house or when your parents take you out to a social event. So having an older sibling in the house, someone with a different intellectual development, at a different stage from where the child is at. So he or she can learn. And having a younger sibling at the same time, the child learns how to adapt and the understanding of having a younger sibling . . . different kinds of exposure.

In other words, Nadra (S$5,000–5,999/month) and Siti Isah (S$4,000–4,999) believed that there may be a set of interpersonal abilities or skills that is integral to being human. Latifa (age 21, Malay, S$6,000–6,999), who said that even "two is too lonely," put it this way: "I think that when you have more siblings maybe you'll be more outgoing, easier to adapt to people." For Wee Leong (age 25, Chinese, S$6,000–6,999), it is also important that such learning takes place in a sibling relationship where "you feel more equal."

Twenty-one year-old Aarti (Indian, S$5,000–5,999) said she wanted two children and shared her own experience that:

> because, we learn that you're not alone, so it's not like only child, we don't learn to be selfish, we always have to consider my sister, consider my brother when we do things. So I think that's how things should be.

Moreover, Aarti had sympathy for children who are the only child in the family:

> In school, sometimes they have to have it their own way, because they don't know what it is to give up or give in to others, because at home, there is no one else to fight for anything with them. And usually their parents will give in to them since they're the only children. But I think when you come from a family with siblings, then you'll know that you cannot always have your own way, you learn to reason out and work things out and not just insist on the way you want to have it.

In sum, focus group interview data show that some respondents desire to have more than one child. Married interviewees highlighted the practical social support that the child may gain from having a sibling and unmarried respondents postulated their ideas about childhood socialization or social and intellectual development— in particular, what they consider to be the positive aspects of a home environment in which siblings can relate reciprocally and communally with each other. These respondents thus articulated a relational-based approach to childbearing and childrearing.

Grooming children for individual competitiveness

On the other hand, respondents also are concerned with raising a child to excel in an increasingly competitive world; they want to "give the best" to their children. Moreover, "giving the best" tends to mean "giving the best education." I first draw on dialogues with married focus group participants to illustrate the link between the cultivation of "individual competitiveness" and childbearing decisions.

Investing resources in a purposeful and planned manner

To begin with, the story of the neighbor of Mr. Krishnan (age 51, Indian, S$4,000–4,999) is instructive. "My neighbor—one [child]. They live in a mansion, just imagine, they live in a mansion, they [can] afford to pay $600,000 over for this house, OK? 'Can't you have another child?'" Mr. Krishnan asked. He went on to share his neighbor's reply:

> They go: "So stressful, spend so much money on them, spend so much time on them." You understand? And the time is not on them [on the child]. It is to prepare them, to prepare them to ensure that they do well in class, well in school, and then in the future, they hope they are someone.

Mr. Krishnan's neighbor is not alone in trying to mold a future "someone." Mr. and Mrs. Owyong, a mild-mannered Chinese couple in their fifties, own a house with a beautiful garden, have a monthly household income of over S$10,000, and have only one teenager daughter Serene. Mr. Owyoung explained what he called "a hidden cost" of raising a child:

MR. OWYONG: You see the kid would actually come and pester you. There's one thing I remember is that her class, her teacher was encouraging them to buy an electronic dictionary, *zhonghwa zi dian*.

MRS. OWYONG: Chinese to English, English to Chinese dictionary.

MR. OWYONG: So everybody was buying it. You cannot [not buy]. Although they say it's optional.

THE ASSISTANT (FRIEND OF SERENE): You feel left out.

Mr. Owyong nodded in acknowledgement and continued:

> Yes and then in class teacher will go through this particular model. So we went ahead to buy, it's not a problem, because we only have one Serene. So, what I'm saying is that this is one of the examples of a hidden cost.

In addition to financial costs, in a separate conversation with Mrs. Owyong, a piano teacher who quit her job to stay at home with her child, and whose timetable is always worked together with the daughter's schedule,[3]further illuminates the demands on parental time:

> I do not want to miss out on her growing up. That's why I make it that even if I'm working, I'm working at home. Even if I'm working, I've a companion that I hire, not the maid. It's a companion that will come in and spend time with her, so that I'm free from her and I can focus on my work, but she is there and knowing that I'm there also.

I was intrigued by the idea of a "companion" and asked, "what do you think it does for the child? Why is it important to have a constant companion?" Mrs. Owyong replied:

> I think it gives her [Serene] a more secure feeling. At the same time, for myself, I know that my child is well and also that her time is not wasted. So right from scratch, I've a timetable planned. Time for play, time to do whatever nonsense. Then time to study, time to read, time to watch TV . . . it's all planned out. Of course there are times when we don't follow the timetable, but it's there. It's there for her to know that there's always a time for everything. I believe that is important.

And, as her husband pointed out, this involves both time and finances. Mrs. Owyong continued:

> Because she's doing a lot . . . three musical instruments. So her fees are a lot. But putting that aside, she doesn't have a lot of tuition. She doesn't travel from one tuition center to another. Most of the time she'll do her own reading or the work that I set her to do. If she watches TV, it's always with a reason . . . When she was young, she was only allowed to watch Chinese shows, not the English shows, to brush up her Chinese. So there's always a motive behind what she does. When she was even younger, when she watched the children's show, even then it was selected by me, that is a good show for her to watch because she'll learn something from there . . . In fact we didn't touch her Edusave in primary school because there wasn't much activities to sign up for. Nothing that attracts me to think that it's worth her time.

This couple may be exceptional in terms of the amounts of resources and time they were able to muster to foster their child's individual talent. Indeed, As Mrs. Owyong tacitly noted, ordinarily, parents give their children tuition classes. At the time of the interview, Serene was going to perform with her orchestra at Carnegie Hall in New York City.

Mr. and Mrs. Lee noted a similar phenomenon among their friends and how it affected their friends' childbearing behavior.

MRS. LEE: She [Mrs. Lee's friend] finds it too troublesome and too time-consuming. And the last thing is money, because she gives the best to her current son. She wouldn't want to spend another bulk of money on another child.

MR. LEE: And we have a couple of friends, who actually because of these considerations are unsure [about having another child]. Because once you have a child, the child is there. You cannot say if you are retrenched or your earning goes down five years later, I don't want this child anymore, just delete that. So quite a few people because of this uncertainty they aren't having kids, and I have a friend who already has a kid and then she realizes that it's such a big commitment, and she's stopping there, and just focusing on that one kid.

And Mr. Lee noted that the expensive cultivation started very young in Singapore, which made the government's pronatalist incentive–a S$150-a-month subsidy for half-day, center-based childcare—seem negligible: "which country in this region charges hundreds a month for preschool, and this is not the most expensive one. Try the Montessori or Pat School House [private preschools], it cost thousands."

While the dialogues above show what the pursuit of individual competitiveness means for parents, what does it mean for the child? Below I report the grandparents—Mr. Palanswami (age 56, Indian, S$4,000–4,999) and Mrs. Palanswami (age 56, Indian, S$4,000–4,999)—observations on competition in their grandchildren's (Senthil, age 8 and Eswari age 7) generation, especially the need for children to have requisite material support to stand equal among their peers.

MRS. PALANSWAMI: My elder son can have one more [child]. One [grandson] is in Primary 1, one [granddaughter] is in K2 [kindergarten 2]. She [the daughter-in-law] can afford to have one more but from what I see, from the way they speak, she cannot have a baby, period. Because they cannot afford it! Nursery school cost you a few hundred dollars a term, a few hundreds you know.

MR. PALANSWAMI: That's a lot of money, and we are not [just] talking about uniforms, [but also] the nitty gritty things that the child wants because the other kids in the class have got it. Those [old] days you did not have to worry. At the most, one clown in the class will have something fancy. If you have a football with you, we will all be friends with you. We will play with the ball, tomorrow you can keep your ball, we will find another one.

MRS. PALANSWAMI: You didn't have to worry. Now, no. [mimicking a child] You have one, I must have one, whether it's tomorrow or next week, I must have that. And the whole class, every kid is like that.

MR. PALANSWAMI: You know they change school bags every other month. They [their grandchildren] know they want a trolley bag, they bring you to the shop and correct you if you make a mistake. They will tell you the brand, they are brand-conscious. So who suffers? The parents suffer. After having two, can they afford it? What will happen is, they will start quarrelling about money.

To illustrate the "individual competitiveness" instilled in children, I further draw on the following exchange between Mrs. Visvanathan (age 48, Indian, a kindergarten teacher) and Mrs. Nair (age 51, Indian, S$5,000–5,999), in which they provide their observations on children and speculate about their cultivation.

MRS. VISVA: Two-years-old girl going to ballet class. Don't even know to sit down. How to stand and dance?

MRS. NAIR: I know someone, the child, you know, she cannot study properly. Piano class, ballet class, bharatanatiam class.

MRS. VISVA: I come across this every week.

MRS. NAIR: How can she concentrate on studies?

MRS. VISVA: But they are intelligent children.

MRS. NAIR: Intelligent but the child is too tired. She goes to all these classes, how can she study?

MRS. VISVA: Every Monday, our conversation time, I will ask this child, the child will say, I took [Bus] 119 from Compass Point to somewhere [for class], the other child will say I went for baking class. Then the other will say "Oh, I went for piano class".

MRS. NAIR: More than the children, the parents [compare]. The parents, "Oh she's sending her children there so I must send my children." Some used to look down on me when I sent my children to PAP [state-funded kindergarten]. I didn't care. They say, oh my child is going to kindergarten there, Baptist kindergarten or Thomson kindergarten [private kindergarten].

As noted earlier, respondents more often than not interpret "giving the best" as "give the best education." Other interpretations do exist, however—in particular, married respondents gave examples ranging from providing the best physical care in the form of "breast milk" to best "standard of living" and meeting "material needs" to mothers staying home to take care of children's emotional needs.

Institutionalized competition in education

The pursuit of "individual competitiveness" reported above may be Singapore's version of the global phenomenon of intensive parenthood and childhood. However, as noted in Chapter 3, the Singapore school system is also hierarchically structured both among and within schools. Among schools, there is a differentiation between "elite" schools and "neighborhood" schools, and all schools are ranked mainly according to academic excellence based on the performance of their students in national examinations such as the Primary School Leaving Exam (PSLE) and the Cambridge General Certificate of Education Ordinary Level ('O' level) and Advanced level ('A' level) examination. Within schools, there are streams: EM1 (or Special stream) with English and "mother tongue" as a first language), EM2 (or Express stream) with the mother tongue as a second language, and EM3 (or Normal stream), which does not emphasize the mother tongue. Thus, competition in favor of getting into the "top" or "best" schools and streams is keenly felt among parents and schoolchildren. This can be seen in the following interview with Mr. and Mrs. Ravindran, an Indian couple in their 50s, and their daughter:

MRS. RAVINDRAN: Here we want our children to go to top school, top this top that. It's all the top things that make parents work even harder and spend all their money on the children. I think it's the way the system is wrong.

MR. RAVINDRAN (with a mischievous smile): I think maybe you're wrong. I think every parent will want to have high aspirations for their children.

MRS. RAVINDRAN: No. because the system is such in Singapore. You don't seem to recognize that. We give our own tuition so that they don't go to the EM3 band [the Normal Stream]. We're banded. It's only now slowly that the minister is taking out the band and everything.

THE CHILD: You have to be first in everything. Even if you're not first but you're good in something else, it's not good enough.

MRS. RAVINDRAN: So every child, every parent wants to go to the best schools. Even now you want to take out the banding of schools you can't!

MR. RAVINDRAN: You already have that stigma.

MRS. RAVINDRAN: Yes! I mean, I want my daughter to go to the best school when she finishes her PSLE, you know what I mean? Every parent. In order to do that, what must you do? To give continuous extra lessons all the time.

At this point of the interview, the sense of having to cope with—and thrive in—a "system" where competition is highly institutionalized is palpable in the family setting. Mr. Ravindran, however, turned to his wife and asked "So you're saying [that] in other countries the parents don't care?" Mrs. Ravindran's telling response is worth quoting at length:

> No, I'm not saying [they] don't care. Other countries they don't have the system where they have top school and bottom school. But I also think it's the affluent society. Because we want to give our kids, we give them everything, and we have to work to give [it to] them . . . We don't think there are poor people in Singapore, I don't think so, compared to third world countries. So, there are different styles, they can accept it but we can't, so we will work and make sure our kids get this and our kids get that. And even though the school fees are low, we as parents want to give our kids the best. Actually it's us who do this to our kids. We want to give them everything, so whether it is swimming classes or [other] lessons . . . But you see also the point, the school system is such that the child who does best will get everything. You know PSLE you get 270 maybe you can go to Raffles [a prestigious secondary school]. You don't get [a high score] you go to these [neighborhood] schools.

This interview poignantly reflects a recurring theme in my findings. First, respondents are aware that they are living within the structural context of Singapore society, in which social mobility rests primarily on educational performance. Second, there is a clear response to institutionalized competition in education—so that "give our kids the best" includes tuition and after-school classes. Third, there appears to be a sense of not being able to do otherwise. In Mrs. Ravindran's case, a hint of reflexivity: "Actually it's us who do this to our kids."

This "giving the best" does not stop at primary schools or secondary schools. As Huey Yee (age 32, unmarried, S$9,000–9,999) said:

> It's too expensive to have a kid. It's too expensive. In Singapore society it's such that without a certificate, you can't go anywhere. Where can you go if you are secondary school graduate? So, every parent's dream will be [for their children] to go to tertiary [education]. So if the child can't make it to National University of Singapore or Nanyang Technological University?[4] You have to send overseas; where would you find the money?

In short, interview data with married couples seem to suggest that the pursuit of "individual competitiveness" involves providing not just the basics but, indeed, all it takes to strengthen the competitive edge of the child. This involves ensuring that the child not only performs well in relation to curriculum demands but develops additional or enhanced capacities beyond what is expected in school. One way to ensure that children can succeed in school is to send them to "tuition" or "enrichment classes"—but in all such cases, additional finances are needed. This has become conventional wisdom even among prospective parents, as seen in Izatti's response (age 23, Malay, S$2,000–2,999):

> I will look at financial and also the education level that I can give to my kids. For me the education concern I would have is not [just] from [the] tertiary [level], it's also from primary school. Because, even though the school fees are quite cheap and everything, there's the supplementary tuition . . . I think education is more important for the kids. So before you reach tertiary you have to have a stable foundation during your primary and secondary life. I was thinking of sending them to Mandarin classes. Since Mandarin is important right now. Just trying to give them what they need for the future.

When I asked Thomas (age 22, Chinese, S$10,000 and over), what would prevent him from having a second child if there was no financial worry, he replied:

> I would think of the competitiveness of the Singapore education system. In the sense that it's too academic-based and not so much holistic education, and, as a parent, you also feel the stress of the kid. I think when your kid goes to school and your kid cannot perform the way that you will like them to, that definitely creates a lot of stress as a parent. If you see one kid struggling already and you have to load this kid up with so much tuition and everything, there's no motivation for you to have another kid, to see the other kid also suffer.

Thus, even when financial measures are presumed to be adequate, what discourages prospective parents from having an additional child is tied to their ideal of providing "the best"—mostly in terms of "the best education"—for the child, and their expectations for the child to perform well, and the stress such expectations might create for the family. Moreover, the expectation is not just for the child to succeed within the exam-based education system, but also to become endowed with cultural capital. In the following interview, the respondent talked about an "enrichment course." Enrichment courses are different from tuition classes, as the former refers to optional and extra-curricular activities such as art, music and sports, while the latter refers to classes that are meant to strengthen the child's performance in compulsory school subjects such as Mathematics, English, and Mandarin. As 22-year-old Chinese university student Jamie articulated:

> I think, before, they [the parental provisions] are easily sufficient, but now every single kid has to go for enrichment courses from young, the parent will have problem thinking of a third child, able to fulfill all the needs. I think that's the barrier.

The issue is not just financial resources, but intangible resources such as parental attention and love. Instead of spreading out resources through having more than one child—hence ensuring that the child at least has one companion—some respondents have decided to have only one child, so that they can "give the best" to the child, as seen in Kamini's (age 21, Indian, university student) reply:

> If we are wealthy, then two is fine. But for me having one kid in just nice, two is like may be a bit more of luxury kind of thing. I don't know, because I think with two kids, your attention is being divided in everything. And like if you do one for one kid, then you have to do it for the other as well. But if you have one kid, you can make sure that the kid is, you can bring up the kid really really well and all the attention and the best have been given to the kid. And having two kids is just like divided attention as well for the kid.

Negotiating between Two Different Perspectives

Focus group discussions provided a platform through which the same individual may be interviewed in different relational contexts and two perspectives may come in direct contact with each other, as the following conversations show. The first is a conversation with Mr. Krishnamurthy (age 57, Indian, landed property), Mrs. Krishnamurthy (age 55, Indian), and their daughter Kamini. Kamini was articulating the ideal of "individual competitiveness," while her parents were explaining how important it was to consider approaching childbearing from an "interpersonal competence" or "companionship" viewpoint.

MRS. KRISHNAMURTHY: One child is not enough. She must have company. My elder one must have company. So, we decided that we have another child.

KAMINI: I want to have one child because it is very difficult to raise the kid in the society now and I want my children to grow up with my friends' children as their companion.

MRS. KRISHNAMURTHY: It won't be the same.

MR. KRISHNAMURTHY: Must have more children. At least two. Minimum two. The minimum two is not only for the country, it is for the relationship . . . for the good relationship . . . and for the companionship and to have more close relationship between siblings involved and for their future after the parents passing away.

In a separate conversation, Kamini stated that she planned to have only one child. Her boyfriend, Kalimuthu (age 22, Indian, S$8,000–8,9999) had kept silent. But when the moderator asked "Don't you think the kid needs a companion?" Kalimuthu leapt in, "Yes, the kid will be really sad." Kamini then explained the crucial role of educational expenditures in her decision-making:

> My concern is the education of the kid. I mean living in luxury is a choice of your own. But education is something that we should give to the kid and to the maximum. Because my concern is that education fee is increasing really tremendously . . . I want the best for the kids and it's like the parents make the decision at the beginning . . . That's why I rather have one than two because I want the best education for my kid. So if I have two, I have to spend double the amount and if the value is going to keep increasing, then I am just going to keep forking out. Honestly speaking, if the education of my kids is going to be settled, I really don't mind having two. Because I have a sister and the companionship is important.

Sometimes, one of the older generation shares the ideals and perspectives of the younger generation, as the following interview with Mr. Nair (age 59, Indian, HDB 5-room) and Mrs. Nair (age 51, Indian) and their daughter Sujata indicates:

MRS. NAIR: When you have more siblings, you know, later stage in life they help one another. Only two [children] means, if anything happens to one child, the other is left alone. I wanted three. But he [referring to Mr. Nair] was very particular about having two.

MR. NAIR: No no no, you see, actually, when I was small, the social status and economic status between the two child family and the five child family was [noticeable]. It is very comfortable for people to sustain with two kids and the small family. They can provide a better standard of life . . . standard of living.

SUJATA: It's true. You [only] have a certain amount of resources. You can only provide so much for your kids and in [the] future if I have children, I want to provide the best for them. I do not want to be put in this position where I'm incapable of providing certain comforts.

MODERATOR: What level of comfort are we talking about?

SUJATA: I'm talking about a good education. I mean these days people are more materialistic, and definitely when my kids go to school, there's this sort of peer pressure for material things. Materialism can come in the simplest objects, even a pencil case. So I don't want my children to be losing out in this aspect. So I want to provide the best for them in all aspects.

In sum, data from the focus group interviews suggests that, although the desire to have more than one child is evident, this is tempered by a conflicting desire to provide abundantly for a child, especially in terms of education. When probed about their comments that "companionship" was an important consideration, each respondent in the following focus group with Singaporean–Chinese university students (Wee Leong, age 25, Chinese, S$6,000–6,999; Michelle, age 22, Chinese, S$5,000–5,999; Chin Kok, age 25, Chinese, S$2,000–2,999) invariably followed up with qualifications.

MODERATOR: Do you think kids would be happier in bigger families?

WEE LEONG: They will have more companions but they will not feel the same, as in you can't give them the best.

MICHELLE: Everyone wants two [children] because of the scenario that they'll be happily playing together or they'll be accompanying each other. Because of the picture in people's mind. We need the two kids to bring up together. But whether you want the second one, I don't know. It's quite a tough choice because of financial concerns. Ideally, we want two, but whether we do two is one thing.

CHIN KOK: Everyone wants two, but you can only afford one.

MICHELLE: Maybe after the first one you really feel you got no time, no money, nothing.

Notice the tendency to bring considerations such as financial and time constraints into decision making, immediately after acknowledging the value of a child growing up with siblings. The argument takes the form "yes . . . , but"—indicating a conflict between an ideal and what they perceive to be a more realistic scenario. The same pattern of what might be called "conditional proviso" in responses is observed repeatedly.

In light of this recurring theme of the need to negotiate between conflicting ideals, we need to understand what tilts decision making in the direction of having just one child or more. I examined the background of respondents of the 29 interviewees (among the 165 individual interviews) who explicitly articulated the rationale for having one or more children in terms of competition and companionship, without influence or persuasion from other individuals. There are suggestive patterns, as Table 6.1 indicates: respondents who are university-educated and from private estate households are more concerned about their children's "competitiveness" relative to "companionship." The data also shows that respondents in "middle-income" households are more likely than their counterparts in upper-income households or lower-income households to emphasize the ideal of individual competitiveness.

Given the limitations of the "non-representative" and small sample size, this pattern nonetheless lends empirical support to Lareau's (2002) argument about class-differentiated childrearing preferences and practices.

Table 6.1 Patterns in respondents' perspectives of the relative importance of individual competitiveness and interpersonal competence

Individual competitiveness or interpersonal competence	*Respondents' educational level*	
	Pre-university	*University-educated*
Total	10 (100%)	19 (100%)
Competition	3 (30.0%)	10 (52.6%)
Competence	7 (70.0%)	9 (47.4%)

Note N=29.

Summary

This chapter attempts to explore childbearing decision-making among citizens as parents and prospective parents in post-industrial Singapore. I delineate two concerns that figure prominently in respondents' decisions to have an additional child: raising a child able to excel in an increasingly competitive world of knowledge-based economies, as well as to raise a child with interpersonal competence—for example, able to relate to and cooperate with others. In line with the first perspective, parents and prospective parents perceive it their duty to create an environment that facilitates a child's academic skills and capabilities, which increasingly includes acquiring "human capital" and "cultural capital" on top of performing well in school. In line with the second perspective, the priority is placed on creating a communal environment that provides a child with familial companionship from a young age and develops the child's moral character in sustaining and navigating social relationships. As the data shows, these two considerations in turn dictate the usage of parental financial resources, energy, and time. In terms of the former, respondents described how they would "give the best" and "give everything" to one child, and the data suggests such giving takes many forms. Moreover, focus group participants noted that children compare activities in which they participate and material goods they possess with one another. The data is thus consistent with the phenomenon of intensification of mothers' and children's lives, as documented in studies in North America (Blackford 2004; Caputo 2007; Chin 2000; Hays 1996; Lareau 2003; Thorne 1999). With the latter perspective, which is so far less noted, which deems it desirable to provide a child with social support and foster interpersonal abilities, this consideration takes priority over and shapes the view of the "limitations" of time and resources needed to raise an additional child.

While it is obvious that individual childbearing decisions involve considerations of financial resources and time, it seems that these two perspectives reflect parents' and prospective parents' concerns about how to make best use of their resources, and the answer lies in their larger "cultural" construction and understanding of which capital better serve a child's interests—the development of a child's "human capital" (for example, individual competitiveness) or "social capital" (companionship and interpersonal competence). This exploratory analysis of the interview data indicates that, in a situation of scarce resources, respondents from wealthier households tend to place more emphasis on the first consideration. Thus, while state policies implemented since the mid-1980s aimed at encouraging parents to have more children by providing an economic bonus, social class differences in decision-making have generated a counter-intuitive result. Although, as Chapter 4 shows, wealthier households seem to stand to benefit more from pronatalist policies that provide financial incentives and family time, it is precisely these parents who are caught in the quest to raise a "gold medalist," having and spending resources to increase individual competitiveness and giving their best in ways they may subjectively feel are never quite enough to secure a guarantee of success.

More importantly, the tendency among individuals from higher-income households to place more emphasis on children's education seems to support the "quantity versus quality theory" in fertility studies. However, upon closer examination, this is not necessarily so. First, "quality" is defined in a rather narrow and one-dimensional way in the extant literature, relating primarily to educational performance. This chapter suggests that social actors themselves have more complex and multifaceted ideas about the "quality"—or more accurately, the "qualities" and "capabilities"—of a child. Both the ability to perform well in school and the ability to relate to others figure prominently in the interview data. This study does seem to bear out the theory's emphasis on the predominance of the former, especially in the case of individuals from middle-income households, in tilting decision-making in the direction of having fewer children. The latter, however, remains largely absent in the theory's notion of quality. Second, the theory posits quantity versus quality as a trade-off. With a multifaceted conception of "quality," however, the relationship between the two is more complex. "Quantity" (i.e. having an additional child in order to provide a sibling) is perceived as a context in which a certain type of quality (i.e. interpersonal competence) can be developed. In short, the relative importance of different human qualities—individual competitiveness or interpersonal competence—is more of a "tough choice" to be worked out, a dilemma to be resolved in childbearing decision-making, whose result cannot be assumed a priori.

7 Conclusion

The relationship between the individual and the state has been theorized extensively in citizenship studies. At the same time, there is an empirical void in our understanding of the institution of citizenship—in Joppke's (2008) words, "what ordinary people associate with citizenship is one of the biggest *lacunae* in the literature." While the chapters in this book deal with seemingly disparate phenomena—biological reproduction, social provisions, national economic development, and state pronatalist population policies—I suggest that they are actually related: "productivism" finds its expression not only in the realm of state welfare provisions but also in state population policies. Moreover, examining social processes involved in the act of "making future citizens" shows competing notions of citizenship seen through the eyes of the state *vis-à-vis* the lived experiences of the individual. Drawing upon 165 personal interviews and 39 focus group discussions conducted in the globalized city-state of Singapore, there is evidence here that the developmental welfare state's overarching emphasis of citizen-responsibility (which simultaneously ensures human resources for the nation's economic development), coupled with population policies that reinforce social inequalities and ignore social diversities, undermine elaborate state policy efforts in encouraging citizens' biological reproduction. To facilitate positive fertility decisions, the state needs to modify the economic production-at-all cost approach and pay much more attention to the increasing importance of citizen–social rights. This suggests that the Singapore government might profitably approach the phenomenon of very low fertility with major initiatives similar to those of other advanced industrialized countries.

In this book, the compulsory, non-redistributive, employers-and-employees-contributed social security system, the Central Provident Fund (CPF), exemplifies the institutionalization of the notion of "citizen-responsibility." As mentioned in Chapter 1, the CPF is a lynchpin or centerpiece in the function of Singapore as a developmental state. The state has deployed the CPF to finance a range of social policies. Loke and Cramer (2009: 1) wrote that "there is much to be learned from the Singapore and CPF experience . . . for national policy efforts in other countries, such as the United States." One of the key features of the "developmental" welfare state is that the state invests in the development of human resources, most notably through education, to enable individuals to participate in the global economy. More importantly, the state expects the individual to be economically productive and responsible for acquiring a wide range of social services for themselves and their immediate family members. The developmental state operates to achieve more "equal opportunities" in terms of education and paid employment for everyone, and at the same time, it sees individuals who fail to participate as reflecting their lack of merit based on the assumption of opportunities provided. The state will come to rescue those who are proven least able to assist themselves.

Lived citizenship and citizens' vision: beyond productivism and toward citizenship–social rights

While the civic-republican model of citizenship, which emphasizes citizen-responsibility, contributes to the rise of Singapore as an "East Asian Miracle" (Hill and Lian 1995), this book reveals that it is only part of a much larger story. As we have seen, in sharp contrast to the state's emphasis on individual self-reliance and familial responsibility, the act of "making future citizens" is perceived by the current generation of Singaporean citizens as a long-term commitment, requiring: more substantial direct state-provided benefits and subsidies; more legal protection of rights; and more supportive institutional arrangements—all of which are lacking at the present.

More direct, substantial, universal and long-term benefits, such as monthly child allowance and home care allowances

One of the most consistent reasons for citizens to say that pronatalist incentives are not encouraging, in addition to the amount being insufficient, is that the Baby Bonus is just short-term benefits. Indeed, it was reported that "the estimated costs for new parents amount to between S$190,000 and S$700,000 to bring up a child to tertiary education level" (Tan, 2010). They view the Baby Bonus as only a temporary form of relief during the first few post-natal years.

Citizens also point out that the work–family-balance policies have yet to recognize the fact that individual life plans are widely variable. Indeed, according to the latest government statistics available, in 2005, while "dual career couples accounted for 44 percent of married couples," the proportion of husband–breadwinner and wife–homemaker remained substantial at 36 percent (Ministry of Community, Youth and Sports). Perhaps more significantly, in that same year, among the 1,025,483 economically inactive residents, 323,086 were self-identified homemakers (Singapore Department of Statistics 2006). In other words, approximately one out of three economically inactive residents was performing "reproductive" work. These citizens who stay home with their children are requesting state recognition of their caring labor through "home care allowances," a provision that has been theorized in the feminist tradition (see Chapter 1).

Legal protection and rights-based notion of citizenship

If the work–family-balance policies were to be more effective, then the government has to be more proactive in regulating and monitoring corporate behavior. For instance, to encourage career-oriented women to consider a child, there needs to be state's legal provision of job security—for example legal protection against dismissal during pregnancy and on grounds of leave of absence. The state also needs to make the workplace accommodate citizens' daily family life, on a long-term basis, through the provision of the right to request flexible working hours, which is available in the British Employment Act or the right to shorter and flexible working hours, which is instituted in the Norwegian Working Environment Act.

Supportive institutional arrangements

Domestic institutions such as education, health and housing are not direct support like a Baby Bonus, but they are indirect support for child development, or human capital formation. More importantly, they are contexts in which citizens consider the possibility of having a child or another child. The requests from citizens for the state to offer free education and free healthcare show that they are no longer able or willing to absorb the financial costs of child rearing. In the view of lower-income and middle-income citizens, subsidized education is insufficient, especially in light of the provision of free public education in other countries, which is in sharp contrast to the slew of miscellaneous fees that they have to pay and the sums they have to spend on after-school private tuition and learning activities in Singapore's highly competitive education system. Indeed, resident household expenditures on these services have increased over the years. For instance, during 1988–2008, monthly household expenditures on housing increased from 17.5 percent to 26.6 percent, expenditures on education increased from 4.7 percent to 5.3 percent, and finally expenditures on healthcare increased from 2.6 percent to 5.1 percent (Singapore Department of Statistics 2003; Singapore Department of Statistics 2009b).

Moreover, with respect to citizens' requests for flexible work arrangement and on-site childcare centers, this suggests that the private sector also has a role to play in the act of making future citizens. That is to say, the private corporation not only has a social responsibility towards a cleaner environment, but also a responsibility towards human reproduction, which requires a more grounded understanding of its employees' family commitments. Indeed, research has also shown that family-friendly policies offer corporations a competitive advantage in employee recruitment and retention (Eaton 2003; Evans 2002; Glass and Riley 1998; Joesch 1997). Finally, citizens suggest specific ways in which the state can encourage more male presence in the family. For example, the state can treat paternity leave provision as the reservist service, give men and women childcare-leave days separately, as well as directly finance such family-leave provisions.

In short, as I have suggested elsewhere, "the state needs to reconsider the economic-production-at-all-cost approach and become more proactive in supporting workers' right to paid employment and family life" (Sun 2009). Will the situation in Singapore shift in the direction of citizen-rights paradigm? The citizens have yet to adopt the language of "entitlement" or individual human rights; they have only spoken of rights in specific contexts—most notably workplace rights. They do, however, request larger and long-term state subsidies for families and suggest that education and healthcare be provided as a public good.

More importantly, such requests for much more substantial state benefits are made in the context of changing material conditions, notably emerging structural unemployment, growing income inequality, and perceived competition from foreigners working in Singapore, as elaborated below:

Structural unemployment and the "asset rich, cash poor" situation

While the CPF assumes full employment, as Chua (2007: 35) pointed out, "structural unemployment has very quickly become a reality in Singapore in the beginning of the twenty-first century." Moreover, "if and/or when unemployment becomes a structural feature of the economy, then the virtuous circle of financial accumulation at household level through public housing homeownership is immediately threatened." In addition, McCarthy *et al.* (2002) noted that because the CPF has stringent de-accumulation rules, it is hard for the workers to get cash out of their CPF accounts. The sense of job insecurity and inadequate financial liquidity was clearly observable in Chapters 4 and 5, particularly among the middle- and lower-income households. Citizens in these households report that such concerns discourage them from considering another child as they are worried about not being able to financially provide for the family.

Growing income inequality

According to the Monetary Authority of Singapore (2009: 2), "the ratio of the average income of the top 20 percent of employed households by income to the lowest 20 percent has risen from 9.99 to 12.15 over the same period [2000–2006]." Verweij and Pelizzo (2009) suggested that:

> despite its high GDPpc (GDP per capita), Singapore's income-inequality profile is in line with those of third world countries. While other affluent Asian nations such as Japan, Korea, and Taiwan have Gini coefficient (a summary measure of income inequality) close to those of European nations (0.25, 0.32, and 0.33 respectively), Singapore's deteriorated from 0.43 in 1998 to 0.47 in 2006—roughly the same as those of the Philippines (0.46) and Guatemala (0.48) and worse than that of China (0.44).

Adjusting for government benefits and taxes, the Gini coefficient was 0.452 in 2010 (Singapore Department of Statistics 2001b).

Moreover, Abeysinghe and Gu (2010: 14) showed that "the lifetime income inequality has been increasing rapidly, especially since the Asian financial crisis. In fact, despite the substantial growth of the economy, the lower income quantile has seen a drop in their real lifetime income." As Chapter 6 indicates, household income can affect children's educational achievements, and parents and prospective parents in this largely middle-income society are limiting childbearing in order to cultivate their existing children's competitive edge in various ways.

Perceived competition from foreigners working in Singapore

The share of foreigners in the employed population has remained roughly unchanged—30 percent—in Singapore between 1997 and 2006. The absolute gains in paid employment by citizens increased during the economic upturn between 2004 and 2006, and "during the economic slowdown from 2001–2003, total employment fell, with foreigners bearing the brunt of the job losses" (Ministry of Manpower 2008). Nevertheless, as Chapter 5 shows, many Singaporeans perceive and experience the presence of foreigners in the work setting as taking away their jobs. Thus, there is relative deprivation on the part of the citizens, particularly when the official data also show that during the decade of 1996–2007, citizens' share of the paid employment declined from 64 percent to 60 percent (the largest share gain was registered in the category of the permanent residents). As noted in Chapter 5, the perceived job insecurity and competition with foreign workers discourage citizens to consider having another child.

Can the Singapore government afford to respond to citizens' requests for larger and long-term state subsidies for families and provision of education and healthcare as a public good? As documented in Chapter 3, the government's finances stood at a surplus of S$24,100 million (approximately US$16,971 million) in 2008, and the Government of Singapore Investment Corp (GIC) manages assets estimated at more than US$100 billion (International Herald Tribune, September 30 2009).

In summary, as the above discussion makes clear, even in a world of highly mobile capital and labor, the state remains vital to the social and economic well-being of its citizens. Indeed, as Midgley and Tang (2001: 245) pointed out, "economic development is meaningless if it fails to bring about significant improvements in the well-being of the population as a whole." In other words, we should see not only increases in welfare expenditures, but also substantial pronatalist incentives for the general public rather than for the selected few.

Making future citizens: lessons for pronatalist policy making

As Myrskyla, Kohler, and Billari (2009: 742) noted:

> the existence of a positive HDI [High Development Index]-fertility relationship at advanced development stages indicates that further development has the potential to reverse earlier fertility declines once countries reach very high HDI levels . . . [.] Specifically, an improved understanding of how improved labour-market flexibility, social security and individual welfare, gender and

economic equality, human capital and social/family policies can facilitate relatively high levels of fertility in advanced societies is needed.

Singapore became an independent nation in 1965 and a "post-industrial" society during the early 1990s. Furthermore, the female labor force participation rate increased from 24.2 in 1965 to 54.3 in 2007. The female labor force participation rate in 2007 was more or less comparable with that of the United States (59.5 in 2008), the United Kingdom (56.1 in 2007), Japan (48.4 in 2008), Australia (58 in 2006), and Switzerland (58.9 in 2008). The total fertility rate reached the replacement level in 1977, and has since declined to 1.62 in 1987, and further down to 1.29 in 2008.

As discussed in Chapter 3, pronatalist concerns have been a top priority in Singapore's public policy making since late 1980s, which entails a multi-pronged approach that the government revisits and fine-tunes on a regular basis. Recent policies instituted since 2000 have included the Baby Bonus scheme and work–life support policies. Housing, healthcare, and education are subsidized in Singapore—80 percent of the citizens and permanent residents live in state-subsidized Housing Development Board (HDB) flats and 90 percent of such HDB flats were "owned" in 2008. There are government-restructured public hospitals and polyclinics and healthcare subsidies for Singaporean citizens that range from 20 percent for individuals with higher-income to 80 percent for individuals with lower income. There is no school fee for the primary-level education and the school fee is only S$60 (approximately US$40) per year for the secondary level. Given this ostensibly favorable environment, it is even more intriguing why citizens, as parents and prospective parents, typically remain unmoved by the pronatalist policy initiatives.

Upon closer inspection, the story is more complex and multi-faceted than is usually reported, namely the rising costs of raising children and the increasing prevalence of dual-income couples. In what follows, I summarize the lessons learned as far as pronatalist population policies are concerned. First of all, it is vital to distinguish between two kinds of pronatalist policy effects: effects on making child-rearing easier versus effects on encouraging childbearing. Citizens in this study applaud various state policies and measures that are making child-rearing easier, and are generally in favor of such measures. However, these policies are not deemed by the citizens sufficient to encourage them to have an additional child. This finding may not be surprising, but it points to an important lesson concerning state pronatalist policies—although policies are couched in the promise of encouraging "childbearing," they are very limited in producing that outcome.

Second, citizens respond to existing policies in varied ways. On the one hand, as many of the semi-structured interview respondents have opined, government policy is making it easier financially for people to raise children. Work–family-balance policies such as extended paid maternity leave are welcomed for allowing parents to spend time with their newborns. Parents are also appreciative of more days of childcare leave that enable them to care for their children when the children fall ill. On the other hand, we have also heard that, for example, pronatalist financial incentives are short term and more like reimbursement and compensation rather than a significant form of encouragement. Work–family-balance policies are not effective because of the lack of job security associated with leave-taking.

The point, however, is not only to note that some policies are deemed encouraging while others are not, but also to explain how and why. How do the responses vary? Generally speaking, family-oriented working women and citizens in the wealthier households tend to regard policies positively. Why? Findings documented in earlier chapters suggest the different responses toward pronatalist policies are a function of:

- the forms in which state benefits are delivered;
- the channels of communication and dissemination of policies; and
- the targeted individuals' combined material position and subjective aspirations.

First, in terms of the existing financial incentives, three out of five respondents mentioned cost of living as a concern—and they, in turn, tended to view financial incentives as insufficient. Moreover, various pronatalist tax rebates and matching funds are perceived to benefit only those with private housing and higher monthly income. As noted in Chapter 4, according to the latest General Household Survey data available (2005), only 15 percent of all Singaporeans reside in private housing and only 20 percent of all resident households have monthly income exceeding S$8000. In addition, while financial incentives are perceived to be biased against homemakers, "work–life support" policies that are designed to provide family time to encourage childbearing are seen as biased against men and career-oriented women—there is no paternity leave provision in the private sector, no legal protection of job security after leave-taking, and parents share the six days of paid childcare sick leave days. This suggests that, ultimately, only a small portion of the dual-earner households (which constitute less than half of all married-couple resident households in 2005) directly benefit from the work–family-balance policies.

Second, the pronatalist policies are communicated primarily through the National Day Rally speeches, government websites, and newspapers. At the same time, as George noted (2010: 261):

> the government can no longer count on reaching the majority of television viewers for its public communication campaigns and key agenda setting messages, such as the Prime Minister's National Day Rally Speech. In 1989, before cable TV and the World Wide Web, half of Singapore's adult population tuned in to watch the National Day Parade on Channels 5 and 8. In 2007, less than one-third did so.

Moreover, access to media channels increases when household income increases—for instance, in 2008, 48.6 percent of the lowest 20 percent household income group had a personal computer in contrast to 93.3 percent of the highest 20 percent. In addition, 40 percent of the lowest 20 percent household income group has internet subscription/access in contrast to the 88 percent of the highest 20 percent. Finally, while households with less than S$1,000 monthly household income spent an average of S$7.7/month on newspapers, households with more than S$7,000 monthly household income spent three times as much—S$21.9/month on newspapers. However, the newspaper expenditures constitute a more significant proportion of household expenditures in the lower income groups than in the higher income groups (Singapore Department of Statistics 2009b). Thus, the dissemination of pronatalist policies, through these channels, privileges the higher income groups. This is in sharp contrast to the communication efforts in the anti-natalist era shown in Chapter 3—"face-to-face motivation continued at the clinics, maternity wards, and homes," and the result was that more than 70 percent of the eligible population were aware of the anti-natalist policy details (Wan and Loh 1979).

Third, the perceived policy inadequacies reflect as much about the policies as the targeted individuals' socio-economic positions and their subjective aspirations. As findings in Chapter 4 show, citizens in lower- and even middle-income households view the pronatalist incentives in the context of rapidly rising prices in state-subsidized flats. This translates into higher down payments, longer periods of housing loan payments and, in some cases, additional CPF interest payments if they use their CPF accounts to pay for the housing loans. In contrast, the issue for the upper-income families is not so much their inability to finance a roof over their head but their own expectation of upgrading to a bigger residence with more rooms. There is also the Housing Development Board's regulation that the applicant citizen's "gross monthly household income must not be more than S$8,000" in applying for the HDB flat. This effectively channels these citizens into the more expensive private housing market.

Citizens at all income levels are concerned with healthcare expenditures, but the nature of their concerns is, again, different. Citizens in lower income households are struggling to pay medical fees at state-subsidized polyclinics and are discouraged by long waiting time. Citizens in middle-income and upper-income households turn to private neighborhood clinics and private hospitals and thus are spending more on healthcare. Indeed, according to the Report on Household Expenditure Survey 2007/2008, "spending on healthcare grew by 5.8 percent per annum between 2002/03 to 2007/08 from $170 to $230. Specifically, there were increases in expenditure on hospitalization, specialized medical treatment, dental services and pharmaceutical products" (Singapore Department of Statistics 2009c). The lowest 20 percent household income group spent 6 percent of their overall monthly household expenditures on healthcare, while the highest 20 percent household income group spent 4.8 percent of their overall monthly household expenditures on healthcare (Singapore Department of Statistics 2009c).

Finally, with respect to education, the interview data show that the miscellaneous school fees for the primary school and secondary schools, seemingly nominal, remain a significant cost for citizens in the lower and middle-income households when considering whether to have another child, while citizens in the upper-income households expect to send their children to private preschool and, ultimately, to the university. They are anticipating high education expenditures. The social pattern of expenditures on education noted in the official national survey is even more dramatic than the expenditures on healthcare: the monthly household expenditure on "education and stationary" ranges from S$115.3/month for the lowest 20 percent household income groups to S$383.6/month for the highest 20 percent income group. Thus, unlike healthcare expenditures, educational expenditures occupy a higher percentage of overall household expenditures for the upper-income families (5.4 percent and above) than for the lower-income families (5.2 percent) (Singapore Department of Statistics 2009c).

In sum, then, it is the interaction between a) market costs associated with child-rearing and b) the parents or prospective parents' class position and their expectations in terms of what they strive to provide for their children, that shapes the effectiveness of pronatalist financial incentives. Similarly, family-oriented women have different reactions toward a paid maternity-leave policy than career-oriented women because of their varying life aspirations. Family-oriented women would not mind quitting their jobs to care for their children while career-oriented women prefer to keep working after childbirth. Thus, legal protection of job security in connection to taking maternity-leave is essential for the policy to be effective for the latter. Most male citizens still perceive their family role to be breadwinners, so leave policy does not figure prominently in their decision-making. However, for men who aspire to be more "hands-on" or to provide their wives with more moral and emotional support through their presence, lament the lack of paternity-leave provisions, particularly in the private sector.

Competing visions of the nation's future

Citizens' perceptions of Singapore's current pronatalist policies reveal a subtle and under-theorized link between notions of citizenship and a classical but subterranean form of positive eugenics. Indeed, one of the most distinctive features of Singapore's three-decade long pronatalist policies is that it is perceived to reinforce, rather than to ameliorate, social inequalities as the state rewards the "economically productive" citizens. In contrast, when pronatalist policies in other nation-states have a bias, they tend to deliver more benefits to the lower-income families, at least on paper (see Chapter 2).

To understand this "exception," one needs to step back in time. As Bittles and Chew ([1998] 2009) noted:

> during the early years of the present [twentieth] century, eugenics was seen as holding the key to future human progress . . . It was envisaged that the eugenic ideal could be pursued in two ways: by restricting the reproduction of persons believed to be of inferior genetic potential (negative eugenics), and conversely by encouraging individuals thought to possess desirable genetic characteristics to increase their fertility (positive eugenics).

There are various routes through which negative eugenics and positive eugenics can be pursued. For instance, Lovett (2007) documented how in the United States in the early twentieth century, Edward Ross and Theodore Roosevelt understood, and used, social and cultural influence to promote selective reproduction. Broberg and Roll-Hansen ([1996] 2005) documented the "negative eugenics" embedded in the sterilization programs in the welfare states in Norway, Sweden, Denmark, and Finland.

The eugenics principle can also be formally coded in population policies; the question is who is restricted and who is encouraged. In Singapore, the positive eugenic "phase" during the mid-1980s when the state encouraged better-educated women to give birth, is well-known and extensively documented. It is also believed to have been discontinued—at least there ceased to be explicit and overt bias based on educational achievement. As the data presented in this book suggest, however, while the eugenic principle may not be explicitly articulated or even consciously intended, differential outcomes and class-aligned support are embedded in the structure of the program implemented since 1987. The current criteria for the restriction and encouragement of reproductive behavior is primarily based on an individual's socio-economic achievement, based on indicators that include but are, not limited to, education, income, property ownership, and employment status. Different elements, such as the forms in which incentives are delivered and the media channels through which information is disseminated, converge to benefit childbearing by citizens of a higher socio-economic status.

In short, it may be suggested that Singapore has a history of "merito-genetics"—based not so much on a now thoroughly discredited ideology of racial and ethnic superiority, but on socio-economic attributes of individual citizens. Again, while these social and economic statuses are typically related to race and ethnicity in multi-racial societies, there need not be any conscious or deliberate intention for policies to target such groups. Such criteria are consistent with the "productivist" principle of the subordination of the social to the economical, and seem to blend seamlessly with the rise of the knowledge-based global economy. Indeed, the state's idea of promoting social reproduction through encouraging individuals of higher socio-economic status to have more children can also be seen through its immigration policies. The granting of permanent residence in Singapore is typically "due to their [the individuals'] economic contributions" (Ministry of Manpower 2008: 3). Moreover, immigrants' family privileges are also tied to the individual applicant's monthly earnings. As Low and Johnston (2003: 219) noted:

> the state has relaxed its immigration policy from time to time to attract the right types of foreign talents and skills . . . a new work pass effective from 1 September 1999 is a graduated one involving three tiers of talents to be attracted.

In essence, the tiers are differentiated according to income levels. Employees on the higher end have the privilege of bringing in their spouses and children as well as their parents and parents-in-law. Skilled workers in the lowest category are not allowed to have their families join them. Thus, there is consistency in the two types of policies—immigration policies and pronatalist policies—that constitute the core of Singapore's population management tools. Both are informed by productivist logic. Such a "merito-genetics" viewpoint, however, blames the poor for their own poverty and ignores the complex political, socio-economic forces and gender relations that shape fertility decisions (Connelly 2008; Luker, 1997).

The extent to which Singaporean citizens imagine a better future for themselves and their families contrasts sharply with the state's meritogenic strategy. As Esping-Anderson (1990) suggested, "the universalistic system [of social provisions] promotes equality of status . . . In this sense, the system is meant to cultivate cross-class solidarity, a solidarity of the nation." Thus, while the state treats the existing inequalities as given and further rewards those in the upper echelon through various pronatalist incentives, the citizens themselves are pointing to a more egalitarian way in which national solidarity can be built upon.

Pronatalist policies as a site for investigating citizenship

Singapore is not alone in its efforts to encourage citizens to have more children. In 2006, the Putin government in Russia introduced its Baby Bonus scheme, offering women who had a second child a cash bonus of 250,000 rubles (approximately US$9,200). In the same year, the Roh government in South Korea announced a large-scale project called "Saeromaji 2010" ("Saero" = new, "maji" = rendezvous) to combat the country's low fertility, which includes its version of the pronatalist policies supporting work–family balance: The government planned to spend a total of US$10.5 billion on the expansion of public childcare facilities, the promotion of parental leaves, and the enhancement of work–family balance during the first five-year phase (2006–2010). In 2009, the city of Shanghai in the People's Republic of China started a public campaign to encourage couples to consider having a second child, even though it has yet to offer any pronatalist financial incentives or start work–family-balance initiatives. These governments are the newcomers joining countries adopting pronatalist policies.

Post-industrial countries are now in the latest stage, at least according to the demographic transition theory. With falling birth rates, coupled with steady death rates, it means population decline, or that population grows only very slowly, in these countries. For several decades, this has led to the formulation and implementation of pronatalist policies, including incentives to encourage citizens to have more children. In Europe, for instance, the French government started the pronatalist policy of "Family Tax Splitting" as early as 1945, a policy in which the tax gains for the third and every subsequent child were double the amount that can be obtained for the first and the second child. The governments in Sweden, Finland, and Denmark instituted monthly children allowance in 1964, 1985, and 2004, respectively. In Canada, the province of Quebec introduced its version of the Baby Bonus scheme in 1988 and the monthly child allowance was established in 1997. In Australia, the family tax benefits started in the late 1970s, and the Baby Bonus scheme was offered in 2002. Japan initiated the "Child Allowance System" in 2000: all children under the age of 3 receive an allowance of 10,000 yen (approximately

US$94). For children aged 3–12, the first and second children receive 5,000 yen (approximately US$47) while the third and subsequent children receive 10,000 yen.

As noted in Chapter 2, the economic model linking income and fertility behavior underlies the pronatalist policies giving financial incentives. The institutional-cultural model treats fertility behavior as a function of the individual's roles, and thus potential role conflicts, in paid employment and in family life. Pronatalist work–family-balance policies usually are aimed at providing individuals with family time to support their balancing act. Because there is little compelling body of research on this topic linking the macro-level state policy with the micro-level individual behavior, the effectiveness of such pronatalist policies is currently subject to debate.

The research reported here suggests that the effectiveness of pronatalist incentives in encouraging citizens' fertility behavior is, in large measure, a function of the citizens' perceptions, knowledge, understanding and interpretation of such policies. Moreover, the important message embedded in citizens' responses toward the existing policies shows that answers to broader questions (such as "What is the nature of government responsibility to its citizens in areas such as healthcare, social security, employment, housing and family benefits?") are likely to determine the effectiveness of pronatalist policy (Sun, forthcoming).

While it may seem a stretch to compare Singapore with Scandinavian countries with a history of social democracy and comprehensive welfare states, it seems that there is nothing intrinsic in the corporatist social insurance and familialism welfare model adopted in continental Europe and East Asia that prevents the state from pursuing a more generous and progressive pronatalist policy suggested by its citizens. In fact, it is already happening in other parts of Asia, most notably Japan, a country also well known for its rapidly declining birth rates, human resources economic development strategy and "developmental" welfare state paradigm. The Democratic Party of Japan was elected with a high voter turnout on August 31st 2009, and broke the incumbent Liberal Democratic Party's 54-year rule. While on the campaign trail, the DPJ pledged to "pay a 'child allowance' of 312,000 yen per annum for all children until they finish junior high school. Make high school education effectively free, and make the university scholarship system much more inclusive" (The Democratic Party of Japan 2009).

Even when the field of pronatalist policymaking gain relative autonomy *vis-a-vis* other state social policies, takes up its share in government budget, and becomes more self-evolving, it is important to keep in mind, as this study suggests, that domestic institutions mediate between the macro-level pronatalist policies and micro-level individual childbearing decisions. That is, when access to education, health and housing is perceived or experienced to be increasingly limited and inequitable—as in the current situation in Singapore—the effectiveness of pronatalist policy initiatives (including both financial and work–family-balance policies) would remain minimal.

Ethnic differentials in total fertility rates and the inherent contradictions in treating citizens as "human resources"

The gap between the aim and outcome of pronatalist policies also reflects an inherent contradiction of the state's human resources economic development paradigm. This study finds that higher-educated female citizens are better informed of the pronatalist policy incentives; however, they are also more likely to be career-oriented women who ideally would like to keep working after having a child, and they are also more likely to limit childbearing because they believe in instilling "individual competitiveness" rather than "interpersonal competence" in their children. In sharp contrast, female citizens with lower level of formal schooling, especially those without university education, are more likely to be completely unaware of the pronatalist incentives; but, they are also more likely to give birth to more than one child because of the belief in developing children's interpersonal competence through sibling relationships. Moreover, they are more likely to be family-oriented women who ideally would like to stay at home or quit their jobs when they have children (even though in reality they may not be able to because of financial concerns).

According to the Singapore Department of Statistics, in 2000, 9.5 percent of Singapore citizens were university graduates, and the proportion of university graduates among the Chinese, Indian, Malay, and "Others" were 10.8, 8.1, 1.8, and 11.0 percent, respectively. Given that there is a higher proportion of university graduates in the Chinese group as compared to the Indian and the Malay groups, one would expect to see a corresponding lower fertility rate among the Chinese group than the Indian and the Malay group, which is the documented ethnic differentials in total fertility rates.

This is not to suggest that group norms or religion explains little of the noted ethnic differentials in fertility. Indeed, group norms and religion shape ideas about the value of children and the relative emphasis of individual competitiveness or interpersonal competence noted in the Chapter 6. However, university-educated Malay respondents discuss their family planning in ways more similar to their university-educated Chinese counterparts than to their less-educated Malay counterparts. This study, therefore, indicates the key role of educational attainment in determining fertility behavior. The fact that women have achieved more formal education over the years, has direct implications for childbearing. As of June 2010, among employed persons aged 15 years and above, 34.7 percent of those with secondary education and above are females (Labour Force Survey of Singapore 2010). The percentage of women in the workforce with tertiary qualifications also rose from 3 percent in 1980 to 11.5 percent in 1997, to 16 percent in 2007, and to 20.6 percent in 2010 (Labour Force Survey of Singapore 2010).

In short, a contradiction exists: an increase in the level of female education contributes to national economic development, but more educated women are less likely to heed the nation's call for increased reproduction. This is precisely because better-educated citizens are more inclined to prioritize their children's "human capital"—that is, place a greater focus on enhancing personal attributes likely to be attractive to future employers—as opposed to a concern for "social capital" (inter-personal social skills) in the form of providing their children with a sibling relationship. But one should not be surprised at such inclinations—after all, the state itself is adopting the "human resources" or the "human capital" approach to economic development. However, one can hardly predict the concerns of employers two decades in the future, and it might turn out that "social capital" will have more cache in the workplace of 2030.

Pronatalist policies as a type of public policy

Towards a more interactive and contextualized public policy-making paradigm

Policy debates are saturated with claims based on a combination of statistical data and putative causal relations between correlations and outcomes. The problem with these claims is that they typically lack any portrayal of the texture and nuance that go into individual decision-making about momentous, life-altering decisions. For example, the outcome of a decision about childbearing is binary: either one has a child, or one does not! However, that decision may have been an agonizing one that could easily have gone either way with just a shift in the balance of the many forces at play—forces ranging from family pressure to career advancement, from the perceived available financial support based on paid employment and/or government subsidies. What appears in gross statistical outcome data as an either/or decision can therefore be deceiving to the policy analyst. However, if we are to better penetrate and discern the context of decision-making, there is an increased chance that altering selected policies can have considerable effect.

The context of post-industrial urban economy engenders lower birth rates that require solutions from the incumbent government of the country in question. Governments cannot coerce or force women to have a specific number of children in order to raise the total fertility rate. If women want to have a certain number of children (and the majority of respondents in this study reported that they would ideally like to have more than one child—see Chapter 6), then the question is: What kind of policies would help?

Interview data indicate that Singapore citizens are attuned to other nation-states' pronatalist policies as they draw comparisons to suggest whether and how the financial and work–life-balance policies in Singapore are (or are not) encouraging. For example, China and Denmark were explicitly named in comparison with Singapore's four-month maternity leave; Germany and UK are used as reference points that employers in Singapore are not as respectful of employees' request for parental leave. It was noted that France provides generous cash benefits to larger families. Interviewees also characterized the Australian government as pro-family in providing monthly home care allowance, sustained education and health subsidies and facilitating reduced work hours. These responses became more serious and intense during focus group discussions when interviewees talked about instances of migration to other countries among family and friends, as well as their own intention to migrate, for reasons related to lack of sufficiently supportive pronatalist policies. In short, as I have suggested elsewhere, globalization enhances citizens' capacity for envisioning the nation (Sun 2010). Nonetheless:

> to the extent that the nation is viewed as a "sentiment of solidarity," its strength depends on how successful the state is in recognizing and negotiating with citizens on the ways in which a particular problem of the "social-collective" should be solved.
>
> (ibid: 2)

More generally, as Liu (2003: 234) argued:

> we need to "bring the state back in"; it does not mean that we treat the state as a vertical, rigid, and authoritarian structure, instead, we should try to understand how the state could manage to strengthen itself through negotiation and interaction with the emerging transnational communities.

The significance of this emerging transnational consciousness is not that the state should always emulate what other countries do. Rather, the point is that unless policymakers know or understand how the policies are actually perceived by *people in the experience*, the policies could be theoretically coherent, but in practice, they can be substantial failures. In other words, the importance of empirical work cannot be exaggerated or over-emphasized in the arena of policy studies.

If, as it turns out, individuals residing in the country in question suggest policy revisions in the direction of other countries' practices, there may be structural (e.g., structural unemployment) and cultural reasons (e.g., the belief in giving children the best education) that prompt similar responses or requests "from the ground." Take, for instance, the issue of the home-care allowance noted in Chapter 5. As Vikat (2004) showed, the Finnish system of monthly home-care allowance succeeded in helping parents through the time before they could go back to work, thus reducing the effect of business cycles on fertility rates. Given the centrality of wages in Singaporean net worth and household wealth, the social security system, and the perceived job insecurity and foreign competition, it is understandable why some citizens are requesting such provisions.

In other words, I have attempted to analyze the relationship between population policies and individual childbearing behavior as a context-dependent social process, an important but often neglected basis for new policy deliberations. Even when governments are increasingly adopting policies that look alike on the surface—most notably Baby Bonus and work–family-balance policies—whether and how these incentives would be effective depends largely on how governments communicate such policies and how people perceive such policies in the course of decision-making. At the regional and global levels, findings of the critical role of contexts or framing should be of interest to policy specialists and analysts of various theoretical persuasions.

Finally, while this research has focused on policies affecting fertility decision-making, it can also be treated as a study of the effects of administrative law. Policies and laws can create, maintain, reinforce, or undermine social hierarchies; they can also acknowledge or ignore social diversities. How they operate and whether they are accepted by the affected individuals and communities are empirical questions.

In this book, on the one hand, citizens' responses toward the pronatalist financial incentives suggest they perceive existing policies as reinforcing the prevailing hierarchy. They suggest that such policies need to be modified to allow for wider access to state benefits. On the other hand, citizens' responses toward work–family-balance policies suggest that existing policies support a "super-mom" paradigm, but they see gender roles are in a state of flux. To be effective, policies need to acknowledge diversity in individual life plans and to respond to both traditional arrangements and ever-developing cultural shifts in citizens' egalitarian aspirations.

Appendix A

Evolution of Singapore's Pronatalist policies (1987–2008)

Policy area	*Pronatalist policies (1987)*	*Policy revisions (2000)*	*Policy revisions (2004)*	*Policy revisions (2008)*
	"Have Three, Or More If You Can Afford It"		"Singapore. A Great Place For Families"	
(A) Monetary Incentives				
A1) Income Tax Relief	(a) *Income Tax Relief, Rebates:* in 1988, tax reliefs of S$750 for the first two children, and S$750 for the third child (increased from S$500). With effect from 1989, relief of S$1500 for the first, second, third, and fourth child.	Unchanged	Unchanged	*Qualifying Child Relief* (QCR) and *Handicapped Child Relief* (HCR): Replacing *Income Tax Relief*—working parents can claim S$4,000 per child for all children under QCR or S$5,500 per child under HCR.
	(b) *Enhanced Child Relief* scheme: Working mothers can claim relief for the first, second, third child, and fourth child of 5 percent, 10 percent, 15 percent and 15 percent of their earned income, subject to S$10,000 cap for each child, criterion for eligibility was 5 GCE O-Level passes.		*Working-mother's Child Relief*: Replaced *Enhanced Child Relief* scheme—Working mothers can claim relief for the first, second, third, and fourth child of 5 percent, 15 percent, 20 percent, and 25 percent of their earned income. The maximum for each child is S$25,000.	*Working-mother's Child Relief*: 15 percent of mother's earned income for first child, 20 percent for second child, 25 percent for third and subsequent child. Maximum claim increased to S$50,000.

	The amount was raised in 1989, to 15 percent, 20 percent and 25 percent of earned income for the second, third and fourth child respectively. The cap was S$15,000 per child.			
A2) Tax Rebates	(a) *Tax Rebate* S$20,000 for the third child in 1987 and extended to the fourth child in 1989. (b) Delivery and hospitalization expenses for fourth child offset against parents' earned income; cap S$3,000.	*Second-child Tax Rebate* offered on a sliding scale for second child born to mother aged below 31, from $20,000 if child was born before age 28 to $5,000 for birth before age 31.	*Parenthood Tax Rebate:* S$20,000 for the third and fourth child, and S$10,000 for the second child. Age requirement for second birth removed.	New *Parenthood Tax Rebate*: S$5,000 for the first child, S$10,000 for the second child and S$20,000 per child for all subsequent children.
A3) Childcare Subsidy	*Childcare Subsidy*: for children of working mothers, S$100/ month for those children who attend full-day childcare for each of the first three preschool children under age 7. Subsidy paid directly to childcare center rather than to parents.	(a) *Infant Care Subsidy*: given to working mothers who put their infants aged 2–18 months in childcare centers (S$150/ month for full-day and $75 for half-day). (b) *Childcare Subsidy for Non-working Mothers:* S$75 subsidy for children of non-working mothers enrolling their children in childcare centers.	(a) Increased *Infant Care Subsidy:* Monthly subsidy for infant care increased from S$150 to S$400 (for full-day). (b) *Childcare Subsidy for Non-working Mothers:* remains at S$75 for non-working mothers who enroll their children.	(a) Increased *Infant Care Subsidy*: Monthly subsidy for infant care increased from S$400 to S$600 for all children. (b) Increased *Childcare Subsidy* (19 months to 7 years old): From S$150 to a maximum of S$300 per month. For non-working mothers, subsidies increased to S$150 per month.

Continued

Appendix A continued

Policy area	*Pronatalist policies (1987)*	*Policy revisions (2000)*	*Policy revisions (2004)*	*Policy revisions (2008)*
A4) Use of Medisave Account (savings in the medical savings account of provident fund savings)	(a) *Medisave for Delivery and Hospitalization Charges*: Payment of delivery and hospital charges for the third child can be made from Medisave account; S$3,000 maximum. (b) *Accouchement Fees for Post-partum Sterilization in Lowe Wards in Government Hospital:* waiver of accouchement fees if post-partum sterilization performed after third or higher order birth.	n.a.	(a) Use of Medisave for maternity purposes extended to fourth child; use for pre-delivery and delivery medical expenses for fifth child onwards provided parents have combined Medisave balance of at leat $15,000 at the time of delivery. (b) Medisave can pay for expenses associated with assisted conception procedures. Withdrawal limit raised from $4,000 to $6,000, $5,000 and $4,000 for the first three cycles.	(a) *Medisave Maternity Package* enables parents to withdraw up to S$450 of Medisave for pre-delivery medical expenses for the first four children.
A5) Maid Levy Relief and Reduction	*Foreign-maid Levy Relief for Working Mothers*: Income-tax relief equal to two times annual foreign-maid levy paid, for working mothers only (year 1990).	Unchanged	*Maid Levy Concession:* Monthly maid levy reduced from S$345 to S$250 per foreign maid for families with children younger than 12 years of age, or elderly persons aged 65 and above. Capped at two foreign domestic maids at any one time.	*Foreign Domestic Worker Levy Concession*: Monthly maid levy reduced to $170 per foreign maid for families with children younger than 12 years of age, or elderly persons aged 65 and above.
A6) Cash Benefits	n.a.	*Baby Bonus* scheme: Two-tier system—(a) Cash gift S$3,000 for the second child and S$6,000 for the	*Baby Bonus* scheme extended to the first and fourth child: (a) Parents receive cash gift S$3,000 each for the first and	*Baby Bonus* scheme: (a) Payout for the first and second child increased to S$4,000. Government contributes up to

		third child over 6 years. (b) Co-savings arrangement Children Development Account (CDA); payable over six years, to be used for childcare or child-development purposes; maximum contribution from the government is S$6,000 for the second child and S$12,000 for the third child. Savings may be used for all children.	second child, and S$6,000 for the third and fourth child each. The cash gift is now given earlier in five installments over a period of 18 months from the birth of the child. (b) The maximum contribution from the government is S$6,000 for the second child and S$12,000 for the third and fourth child.	S$6,000 to the CDA for the first and second child. The cash benefit for the third and fourth child remains unchanged at S$6,000. The government's CDA matching contribution is capped at S$12,000 each for the third and fourth child. The fifth child and beyond are not eligible for cash grants, but the government will have a matching contribution of up to S$18,000 for the fifth child and beyond.
A7) Grandparent Caregiver Relief	n.a.	n.a.	Working mothers can claim relief of S$3,000 if their parents or parents-in-law look after their children below age 12.	Unchanged
Non-monetary Incentives				
(B) Housing				
Public Housing	*Public Housing Upgrading for Three-child Families:* The rules were altered to make it easier for families with a third child to sell their three-room or larger apartment and buy a bigger one.	*Public Housing for Newly-weds:* Down payment for the purchase of a four-room flat can be made in two stages, 10 per cent when signing the agreement and the other 10 percent when taking possession of the apartment.	*CPF Housing Top-Up Grant for Singles Getting Married*: Singles who previously received Government-housing grant may apply for top up to quantum given to couples if they decide to marry.	*Third Child Priority Scheme:* Families with more than two children will be included in the first balloting round for HDB. 5 per cent of available flat supply is set aside for this scheme. HDB Top-Up Grant remains.

Continued

Appendix A continued

Policy area	*Pronatalist policies (1987)*	*Policy revisions (2000)*	*Policy revisions (2004)*	*Policy revisions (2008)*
(C) Education				
Primary School Registration	Priority for children from a one-child, two-child, or three-child family. Disincentives against third and higher order births removed.	Unchanged.	Unchanged.	Unchanged.
(D) Work–Family Balance				
D1) Public Sector Flexible Work	*Part-time Work for Female Civil Servants*: women officers in the civil service with a child below 6 years of age can convert their full-time job into part-time work (21 hours per week) up to a maximum of 3 years at half-monthly salary.	*Flexible Work for Government Departments:* An officer can work five days per week but needs to work long hours during the five days to clock a total of 42 hours. The departments must still operate a six-day week.	n.a.	n.a.
D2) Public Sector Leave	(a) *Childcare Leave for Female Civil Servants*: Up to four years unpaid leave to care for young children, subject to exigencies of service. (b) *Sick Childcare Leave for Female Civil Servants:* Working mothers can apply for five days of paid unrecorded sick childcare leave for each child under age 6 for the first three	(a) *Paid Marriage Leave:* A government employee can take three days' paid marriage leave when getting married for the first time. (b) *Paternity Leave for Civil Servants:* Fathers in civil service can take three days' paternity leave for the first three children.	n.a.	n.a.

	children (total 15 days annually). (c) *Unrecorded Sterilization Leave for Civil Servants*: Eligibility for one week unrecorded post-sterilization leave restricted to those with no O-Level passes.			
D3) Paid Maternity Leave	n.a.	Working mothers can take eight weeks of *Paid Maternity Leave* for the first three children (previously available only for the first two children). Paid by Government (rather than employer), cap at S$20,000.	(a) *Paid Maternity Leave*: Extended to working women giving birth to their fourth child. Leave period lengthened from eight weeks to twelve weeks for the first four births. (b) Four weeks' maternity leave for adoptions, to be paid by Government and capped at S$10,000.	*Paid Maternity Leave*: Increased from twelve to sixteen weeks. The first eight weeks are paid by the employer, and the subsequent half is paid by the government at a S$20,000 cap. The full sixteen weeks are paid for by the government for the third and subsequent confinement, capped at S$40,000.
D4) Paid Childcare Leave	n.a.	n.a.	*Statutory Childcare Leave:* Two days of employer-paid childcare leave for each working parent with children under age seven.	Paid childcare leave increased to six days for both working parents.
D5) Five-day Workweek for Civil Servants	n.a.	n.a.	A shift from a five-and-a-half-day workweek to a five-day workweek in the civil service, but the total number of hours for every employee remains at 42.	Unchanged

Continued

Appendix A continued

Policy area	*Pronatalist policies (1987)*	*Policy revisions (2000)*	*Policy revisions (2004)*	*Policy revisions (2008)*
D6) "Work-Life Works!" Fund	n.a.	n.a.	S$10 million fund. All private sector organizations can apply for grants from the fund to defray the cost of introducing measures that can help employees to better achieve work–life harmony.	Unchanged
D7) Unpaid Childcare Leave	n.a.	n.a.	n.a.	Unpaid childcare leave for both working parents introduced. Each parent receives six days a year for children below age 2.
D8) Maternity Protection	n.a.	n.a.	n.a.	Employer will be required to pay for maternity leave benefits if employee is: (a) dismissed without sufficient cause within the last six months of pregnancy, or (b) retrenched within the last three months of pregnancy.
(E) Other Initiatives				
Counseling	(a) *Abortion Counseling*: Compulsory pre- and post-abortion counseling for secondary educated women with fewer than three children.	n.a.	n.a.	n.a.

	(b) *Pre-sterilization counseling*: Compulsory counseling for men and women with only one or two children.			
Equal Medical Benefits	n.a.	n.a.	Female employees in the civil service are allowed to claim medical benefits for their husbands and unmarried children under the age of 18.	n.a.
Fertility Treatment	n.a.	n.a.	n.a.	*Government Co-Funding for Assisted Reproduction Technology*: Government will co-pay fertility treatments for women below the age of 40 at public hospitals. It will fund half the cost up to S$3,000, for a maximum of three cycles per Singaporean couple.
Social Development Units	*Social Development Unit* (SDU): Established in 1984 to provide opportunities for social interaction and match-making services to single officers in government departments, statutory boards, and government-linked companies that employ university graduates.	n.a.	n.a.	*Social Development Unit* (SDU) and *Social Development Service* (SDS) to be merged.

Source:
Adapted from Yap 2009.
Ministry of Community Development, Youth and Sports 2008.
http://fcd.ecitizen.gov.sg/MarriageNParenthoodPackage/

Appendix B

Survey on marriage and having children in Singapore

STRICTLY CONFIDENTIAL

Name of the interviewer: ________________________
Date: __________________(DD/MM/YY)
Time at the start of the interview: _____:_____ ❑ AM
❑ PM

Student announcement to interviewee:

In this survey, we are interested in understanding what Singaporeans think about marriage and having children. This is a NTU (Nanyang Technological University) research project. We appreciate your help in answering our questions according to your personal views. Our researchers guarantee the confidentiality of information from all questionnaires. The information you provide will be used for research purposes only.

Section A: Value of children

1 Do you have any children?
❑ Yes
❑ I am expecting my first child
❑ No

If <u>**YES**</u>,

1a) How many do you have? _________
❑ ______ boys; ❑ ______ girls)
[Interviewer: Tick if respondent is expecting next child]

1b) Could you please tell me what your reasons are for having a child/children?

____

____

____

____
____

If **NO**,

1c) Do you think you will have a child/children in the years to come?
- ❑ Yes
- ❑ No

1d) What are your reasons for having/not having children in the years to come?

____
____
____
____
____
____

2 If you could have any number of children you want, how many children do you want?

________ number of children
________ no children **[Skip to 2c]**
________ don't know **[Skip to 2c]**
________ no preference **[Skip to 2c]**

2a) Of these, how many boys would you like to have? How many girls?

_____ boys; ______girls **[Interviewer: Probe why]**
_____ boy or girl doesn't matter
[Interviewer: Probe]____

2b) If you have a child/would like to have a child, your ideal/best choice is to:
- ❑ not work before and after having a child/children
- ❑ keep working after having a child/children
- ❑ quit your job after having a child/children

2c) In the years to come, how many children do you think you will be likely to have?

______ children _____ Don't know

2d) Of these, how many boys and how many girls would that be?

______ at least one boy; ______ at least one girl **[Interviewer: Probe why]**
______ don't know
[Interviewer: Probe]____

3 For young children, up to 3 years old, who do you think is best to look after them?
(choose one)
❑ By myself
❑ By my husband/partner
❑ By my parents
❑ By my parents-in-law
❑ By other relatives; please specify ______________________________
❑ By maid/nanny/babysitter; other **paid help**, please specify
____
❑ Daycare center
❑ Others; please specify______________________________

[Interviewer: Now, let's talk about job and marriage.]

Section B: Marriage and employment

4 Have you ever been married?
❑ Yes
❑ No

4a) If **YES**, what is the age you were first married? ________

4b) What is your current marital status?
❑ Married
❑ Separated
❑ Widowed
❑ Divorced
❑ Re-married

4c) If **NO**, at what age would you like to get married?
❑ Does not want to get married **[Skip Q5]**
❑ Don't know
At age_______

5 After marriage, your ideal/best choice is to:
❑ keep working after marriage
❑ quit your job after marriage

6 Now, may I ask about your current living arrangement?

6a) How many people are you now living with? ___________ persons

6b) Who are they? Is this living arrangement temporary (i.e. only for less than six months) or permanent (i.e. for more than six months)?

	Temporary	Permanent
❑ Husband/spouse/partners		
❑ Children		
❑ Father		
❑ Mother		
❑ Mother-in-law		
❑ Father-in-law		
❑ ____ brothers ____ sisters		
❑ Spouses of brothers and sisters		
❑ Father's father		
❑ Father's mother		
❑ Mother's father		
❑ Mother's mother		
❑ Step-father		
❑ Step-mother		
❑ Spouses of parents (Father/Mother)		
❑ Others; please specify ________________		

[Interviewer: Skip Questions 7 & 8 if the interviewee does not want to get married.]

7 What is the best/ideal living arrangement for you after marriage?
❑ My husband
❑ My/our children
❑ My father
❑ My mother
❑ My father-in-law
❑ My mother-in-law
❑ Live-in maid
❑ Others; please specify ____

8 According to your parents, after marriage, what kind of living arrangement is best?
❑ My husband
❑ My/our children
❑ My father
❑ My mother
❑ My father-in-law
❑ My mother-in-law
❑ Live-in maid
❑ Others; please specify ____

[Interviewer: Now let's talk about what is done for the families in Singapore.]

Section C: State policies

9 **For respondents with children: [Skip to Question 10 for respondents without children]**
Was there anything the government did that helped you decide to have a child/children?
❑ Yes
❑ No

9a) If you are deciding whether to have another child, is there anything the government can do that will help you decide?

____
____
____
____
____
____
____
____

10 **For respondents without children:**
If you are deciding whether to have a child, is there anything the government can do that will help you decide?
❑ Yes
❑ No

10a) Probe: ________________________________
____
____
____
____
____
____
____

11 How many children do you think the Singapore government wants each couple to have?
______ number of children
______ the more the better
______ it depends; please specify ________________
______ don't know

12 As far as you know, has the government done anything to **help families** in Singapore?

❑ Yes

❑ No **[Skip to 12b]**

12a) If **YES**, can you please tell me what the Singapore government has done?

____

____

____

____

____

12b) If **NO**, what do you think needs to be done by the government to help families?

____

____

____

____

____

13 As far as you know, is there any government policy that **encourages people to have more children**?

❑ Yes

❑ No **[Skip to 13d]**

13a) If **YES**, can you please tell me what these policies are?

____

____

____

____

____

13b) Which policies do you think actually work? **[Interviewer Probe: In what ways?]**

____

____

____

____

____

13c) Among these policies, which one(s) do you think are **NOT** working? **[PROBE]**

13d) If **NO**, what needs to be done by the government in terms of policies to encourage people to have more children?

14 **What is it that you need in order to have the number of children you want [interviewer refers back to Q2]?**

15 Is the government making it easier **financially** for people to have more children?

❑ Yes

❑ No **[Skip to 15b]**

15a) If **YES**, can you please tell me what the government is doing?

15b) If **NO**, can you tell me how the government can make it easier, financially, to encourage people to have more children?

16 Among your friends and family members, was there anything that the government did to help them decide to have a child/children?

17 Among the existing family policy incentives, could you tell me if you know or have used them:

	I know of and I have used	I know of but have not used	Unaware
Cash benefits			
Childcare subsidies			
Income tax rebates			
Housing allocation			
Housing subsidies			
Maternity leave			
Primary school registration			

18 Among the existing policy areas, could you rank their importance for encouraging families in general to have more children:

	Not important at all	Not very important	Important	Very important
Cash benefits	1	2	3	4
Childcare subsidies	1	2	3	4
Income tax rebates	1	2	3	4
Housing allocation	1	2	3	4
Housing subsidies	1	2	3	4
Maternity leave	1	2	3	4
Primary school registration	1	2	3	4

19 Do you think policies providing old age support and Medicare in the Central Provident Fund (CPF) scheme would affect your decision to have or not to have children?

____

____

____

____

____

20 Among your family members and friends, who has an opinion for whether to have or not to have children?

____

____

____

____

____

21 Among those who have opinions, whose opinion is the most important and whose opinion is less important?
[Interviewer: List from the most important to the least important. 1 = the most important; 2 = less important; 3 = even less important. . .]

____

____

____

____

____

22 Among your families and friends, who do you think SHOULD have the most say in your decision to have or not have children?"

____

____

____

____

____

[Interviewer: To put your answers in context, we'd like to gather some background information from you.]

Section D: Respondent's background

23 Name: ____________________________

24 Please tell me which year you were born? __________

25 What is the highest educational qualification you have attained?
❑ No formal qualification/lower primary
❑ Primary
❑ Secondary
❑ Upper Secondary
❑ Polytechnic Diploma
❑ Other Diploma and Professional Qualification
❑ University

26 What is your ethnic group?
❑ Chinese
❑ Malay
❑ Indian
❑ Other ethnic group; please specify: ______________________________

27 What language do you usually speak at home?

28 What is your religion?
❑ Buddhism
❑ Islam
❑ Taoism
❑ Hinduism
❑ Christianity (❑ Protestant; ❑ Catholic)
❑ Other religion; please specify___________________________________
❑ None

29 What is your household type:

❑ HDB flats – ❑ 5 room
❑ 4 room
❑ 3 room
❑ 2 room
❑ 1 room
❑ Executive condominium/flats
❑ Others
❑ Other public flats
❑ Condominiums and private flats
❑ Landed properties
❑ Others; please specify

30 Are you currently:

❑ working
❑ not working but have actively been looking for work during the past 6 months
❑ not working in a job and have not looked for a job for the past 6 months
❑ housewives
❑ students
❑ students with part-time jobs
❑ retired
❑ disabled
❑ others; please specify:______________________________

31 If you are currently working (for income), what is your occupation?

❑ Senior officials and managers
❑ Professionals
❑ Associate professionals and technicians
❑ Clerical workers
❑ Service & sales workers
❑ Agricultural and fishery workers
❑ Production craftsmen and related workers
❑ Plant and machine operators and assemblers
❑ Cleaners, labourers, and related workers
❑ Workers not classifiable by occupation

32 If you are currently working, are you:

❑ Employer
❑ Self-employed
❑ Employee
❑ Unpaid family business worker

33 What is your general mode of transportation?

____

34 Are your mother and/or father still working (for income)?
❑ Yes
❑ No **[Skip to D12c and D12d]**

35a) If YES, what is your father's occupation?

35b) If YES, what is your mother's occupation?

35c) If NO, what was your father's occupation?

35d) If NO, what was your mother's occupation?

36 What was/is the highest educational qualification your father has earned?
❑ No formal qualification/lower primary
❑ Primary
❑ Secondary
❑ Upper Secondary
❑ Polytechnic Diploma
❑ Other Diploma and Professional Qualification
❑ University

37 What was/is the highest educational qualification your mother has earned?
❑ No formal qualification/lower primary
❑ Primary
❑ Secondary
❑ Upper Secondary
❑ Polytechnic Diploma
❑ Other Diploma and Professional Qualification
❑ University

Family's financial status

38 Is the home you are currently staying in owned by you, by your parents, parents-in-law or by someone else?
❑ Owned by respondent
❑ Owned by respondent's spouse
❑ Owned by respondent and her spouse
❑ Owned by parents
❑ Owned by parents-in-law
❑ Owned by someone else

39 What is the total monthly household income from work? (include the sum of income received by all members of the household from employment and business)

❑ Below 1,000
❑ 1,000–1,999
❑ 2,000–2,999
❑ 3,000–3,999
❑ 4,000–4,999
❑ 5,000–5,999
❑ 6,000–6,999
❑ 7,000–7,999
❑ 8,000–8,999
❑ 9,000–9,999
❑ 10,000 & over

40 How many adults and how many children (under 15) depend on these sources of income?

❑ adults (including the respondent) ❑ child(ren)

41 Is your family's income enough to pay your family's current level of expenses? Is your family's income more than enough to cover expenses, just enough, not quite enough or not at all enough?

❑ More than enough
❑ Just enough
❑ Not quite enough
❑ Not enough at all

42 If you are currently working (for income), what is your personal monthly income?

❑ Below 1,000
❑ 1,000–1,999
❑ 2,000–2,999
❑ 3,000–3,999
❑ 4,000–4,999
❑ 5,000–5,999
❑ 6,000–6,999
❑ 7,000–7,999
❑ 8,000–8,999
❑ 9,000–9,999
❑ 10,000 & over

43 In the past 12 months, did you give money to your parents?

❑ Yes; What is the approximate percentage of your household income?

____

❑ No

44 In the past 12 months, did you receive money from your parents?

❑ Yes; What is the approximate percentage of your household income?______________

❑ No

45 When you (and your husband/partner) are old, from what sources do you hope to get income or support for your living expenses? From a business, property, farm, savings, pension, sons or daughters, or other sources? **[Read each of the following sources aloud.]**

❑ Business income

❑ Property/real estate income (sale, rent)

❑ Savings or interest on savings

❑ Pension, severance pay

❑ Other sources; please specify:_______________________________________

❑ Son(s) **[If mentioned son(s), ask D22b. If not mentioned, ask D22a.]**

❑ Daughter(s) **[If mentioned daughter(s), ask D22d. If not mentioned, ask D22c.]**

46a) You did not mention your son(s) as an income source. Do you hope **NOT** to depend on your son(s) at all financially? Or, do you hope to depend on him/them for only a small amount of your income, or for most of your income?

❑ 1 Hope not to depend on son at all financially

❑ 2 Hope to depend on son for only a small amount of financial support

❑ 3 Hope to depend on son for most of financial support

❑ 4 Not sure

46b) You mentioned your son(s) as an income source. Do you hope to depend on him/them for most of your income or for only a small amount of your financial support?

❑ 1 Hope to depend on son(s) for most of financial support

❑ 2 Hope to depend on son(s) for only a small amount of financial support

46c) You did not mention your daughter(s) as an income source. Do you hope **NOT** to depend on your daughter at all financially? Or, do you hope to depend on her for only a small amount of your income, or for most of your income?

❑ 1 Hope not to depend on daughter at all financially

❑ 2 Hope to depend on daughter for only a small amount of financial support

❑ 3 Hope to depend on daughter for most of financial support

❑ 4 Not sure

46d) You mentioned your daughter(s) as an income source. Do you hope to depend on her/them for most of your income or for only a small amount of your financial support?
❑ 1 Hopes to depend on daughter(s) for most of financial support
❑ 2 Hopes to depend on daughter(s) for only a small amount of financial support

This concludes the interview. Thank you very much for your help!!

Interview ending time

Time: _________: __________ ❑ AM
❑ PM

Appendix C

Components of the CPF system

Purpose	*Program*	*Year Introduced*
Home Ownership	Approved Housing Scheme	1968
	Approved Residential Properties Scheme	1981
	Middle-Income Housing Scheme	1975
	Use of Special Account Savings for Housing Installments	1999
Investment	Singapore Bus Services (1978) Ltd Share Scheme	1978
	Approved Investment Scheme	1986[a]
	Approved Nonresidential Properties Scheme (ANRPS)	1986
	Share-Ownership Top-Up Scheme (SOTUS)	1993
	CPF Investment Scheme	1997
	CPF Investment Scheme—CPFIS-SA	2001
	New Singaporean Shares (NSS)	2001
	Economic Restructuring Share (ERS)	2003
Insurance	Home Protection Insurance Scheme	1982
	Dependents' Protection Insurance Scheme	1989
	MediShield Scheme	1990
	MediShield Plus	1994
	MediShield Scheme for the Elderly (MSE)	2000
	ElderShield	2002
	Private Medical Insurance Scheme (PMIS)	2005
Others	Company Welfarism through Employers' Contribution (COWEC) Scheme[b]	1984
	Medisave Scheme	1984[c]
	Minimum Sum Scheme	1987
	Topping-up of the Minimum Sum Scheme	1987
	Financing of Tertiary Education in Singapore	1989
	Edusave Scheme	1992
	CPF Top-Up Scheme	1995
	Pre-Medisave Top-Up Scheme	1995
	Medisave Top-Up	1997
	Special CPF Top-Up Scheme	2000
	CPF LIFE	2009

Source:
Central Provident Fund (2005b)

Notes:
[a]From October 1, 1993, divided into Basic and Enhanced investment schemes.
[b]Present status for this scheme is unclear.
[c]From 1994, self-employed persons must contribute to the Medisave system

Notes

1 Introduction: making future citizens

1 Kim (2000: 8) notes that global trade has continued to expand as a proportion of world GDP. Trade GDP ratios increased to 5–20 percent—even higher for some developed countries—compared with around 12–13 percent for advanced industrialized countries during the gold-standard era. Notably, the volume of international merchandise trade in 2000 was sixteen times what it was in 1950. In addition, Kim states that national economic activity has increased by as much as one-third. The service sector, for instance, has more than doubled in the past decade to more than US$1 trillion annually.

2 According to the International Labour Organization (2006), international migration figures more than doubled between 1975 and 2000, from a total of 75 million people living and working outside their homelands to well over 150 million. The ILO estimated that 86 million of the 175 million migrants in the year 2000 were migrant workers.

3 According to Kim (2000), global financial flows have expanded more rapidly than world trade or income, with daily turnover in foreign-exchange markets rising from US$15 billion in 1973 to US$820 billion in 1992, and US$1.5 trillion by 1998. The volume of international banking transactions increased from US$265 billion in 1975 to US$4.2 trillion in 1994. Current globalization of finance capital is more extensive and intensive than during the gold-standard era. In addition, Kim states that global FDI inflows and outflows were at US$463 billion and US$475 billion respectively in 1997, nearly twice what they had been in 1990, and some sevenfold their volume in 1980.

4 The United States' per capita GDP was US$47,284 in 2010 (International Monetary Fund 2011).

5 According to "Glossary: Census 2000 Concepts and Definitions,"

> Singapore citizens and permanent residents are classified as Singapore residents or the resident population. Singapore permanent residents refer to non-citizens who have been granted permanent residence in Singapore. Non-resident population are those who are non-citizens and non-permanent residents of Singapore, such as employment pass holders, work permit holders, student pass holders, dependent pass holders and long-term social visit pass holders (Singapore Department of Statistics 2000a).

6 As Daly (2010: 6) articulated, "welfare . . . refers to a set of ideals and practices characterising human behaviour across a variety of sites: state, family, community, market . . . [.] Welfare has to be located as a part of a system of social and institutional relationships through which a collective infrastructure and set of social arrangement is put in place."

7 Chang (2010a: 444) defined "compressed modernity" as "a civilizational condition in which economic, political, social and/or cultural changes occur in an extremely condensed manner in respect to both time and space, and in which the dynamic

coexistence of mutually disparate historical and social elements leads to the construction and reconstruction of a highly complex and fluid social system."

2 Low fertility and pronatalist population policies

1 Marriage remains as a precondition for childbearing in these countries; therefore, delayed marriages or non-marriages is closely linked to fertility rates (Jones 2007).
2 Available at www.nptd.gov.sg

3 Economic development, social investments, and population control

1 Chua and Tan (1999) "Where the New Middle Class Sets the Standard" in *Culture and Privilege in Capitalist Asia*. M. Pinches (ed). London: Routledge.
2 At the time of writing, Singapore held the most recent General Election on May 7, 2011. Mydan reported in the *New York Times* that "the ruling People's Action Party led by Prime Minister Lee Hsien Loong was returned to power on Sunday with a majority of 60 percent of the vote after a hard-fought parliamentary campaign in which opposition parties made their strongest inroads since Singapore's independence in 1965." (Mydan 2011).
3 At the top of the scale, Class A wards give patients their own room and all-frills service. The daily ward fee, not subsidized at all by the state, is S$135. Government subsidies then operate on a sliding scale for Class B1 (20 percent), B2+ (50 percent), B2 (65 percent), and C (80 percent) wards. As the subsidy rises, quality of service falls. In Class C wards, there are at least eight beds, no air conditioning, and no frills.
4 The last digits do not add up—these are numbers in the original publication (Singapore Department of Statistics 2001).

4 Class-differentiated pronatalism

1 Focus group #35 Mr. Palanswami (Indian, age 56, S$4,000–4,999):

> They've got to change . . . giving free education to Singaporean citizens. Now education is more or less compulsory, right? You have to send your child to school, otherwise they come around and ask you why. But do they from the very start say you have to send your child to school, you don't have to pay? Why can't they say that?

Focus group #28 Mr. Krishnan (Indian, age 51, S$4,000–4,999): "As I said again, it's not just financial subsidies, but it is for long-term financial subsidies . . . Because, as I said again, you [the government] put so much emphasis on education, it's not free."

Mr. Balasingam (Indian, S$4,000–4,999):

> The primary reason is the financial aspect of it. I think the government can do more by providing free education. From preschool to university . . . As in, say, countries like the UK, Australia . . . OK, as long as you're a citizen, they provide this for you . . . Even if you [the government] don't give [free] tertiary [education], that's fine. I want free education from the time the child is born, at least until pre-tertiary . . . OK, if you think policy does not allow free tertiary education, fine. But basics as a parent, what will I think of first? The basics for my child must be covered. He must have a basic education, he must have a basic health care.

Focus group #9, Kathleen (Chinese, age 31, S$10,000 and above) and Huey Yee (Chinese, age 31, S$9,000–9,999):

HUEY YEE: A lot of my friends, they are like trying to get PR [Permanent Resident status] in Australia, because they know that if the child is born there, education is free till tertiary. That's like a big load off a parent's mind, I think.

KATHLEEN: Ya. Free education maybe they just give you up to secondary school. Maybe JC [junior college].

2 Focus group #23, Mrs. Wong (Chinese, age 27, executive HDB apartment, S$6,000–6,999): "Free education. University education is a big concern."

3 Specifying economic contexts in which the financial incentives are perceived and responded to by citizens may be more important than it seems if we take into account what macroeconomists have noted of the relationship between inflation and unemployment rates—in particular, the Phillips curve. As Bade and Parkin (2007) explain, "the short-run Phillips curve presents a trade-off between inflation and unemployment because, along a given curve, a lower unemployment rate can be achieved only by paying the cost of a higher inflation rate, and a lower inflation rate can be achieved only by paying the cost of a higher unemployment rate." In other words, the ideal scenario of low inflation and low unemployment seems theoretically impossible according to the rules of macroeconomics. This suggests that governments' pronatalist financial incentives need to be fine-tuned to the predominant larger economic context in order to be effective.

6 Constructing children's multi-dimensional qualities

1 Focus Group #24: When the moderator asked "Why do you want to have four? Is there a reason?" Ms. Lee (age 36, Chinese, S$10,000 and over) replied, "I don't like to have one child because I think it's very lonely. I just thought that actually for our children, it's good to have siblings other that just by themselves or you know it's just one more person, he [referring to her husband] came from a two-child family." Mr. Lee (age 36, Chinese): "So it's pretty boring and lonely childhood." Other examples, focus groups #2, #6, #9, #10, #25, #28, #29, #33, #34, and #36.

2 Focus group #17 (Ismail). In addition, Sukifli (age 24, Malay) said, "During [family] occasions I mean everybody, just more people around . . . [It is] noisier. In a good way." Focus group #7 Jamie (age 22, Chinese), made it a point to say that her experience in growing up as an only child is "Why I believe in not having not just one kid, but realistically, circumstances will make me think that two will be enough, definitely not one, but at least two and to see how it goes around, to see if that I can even have three."

3 Mrs. Owyong: "My timetable is always working together with my daughter's timing."

4 The only two comprehensive universities in Singapore.

Bibliography

Abeysinghe, T. & Gu, J. (2010) Lifetime income and housing affordability in Singapore, *Urban Studies*, 48(9), 1–17.

Ahlburg, D. A., Kelly, A. C. & Mason K. O. (1996) *The impact of population growth on well-being in developing countries*, Berlin, New York: Springer.

Akdere, M. (2005) Social capital theory and implications for HR development, *Singapore Management Review*, 27: 1–24.

Alwin, D. F. (1991) Family origin and cohort differences in verbal ability, *American Sociological Review*, 56: 625–638.

Anderson, B. (2004) Unintended population consequences of policies, *Population and Environment*, *25*(4): 377–90.

Andersson, G. (2008) A review of policies and practices related to the "highest-low" fertility of Sweden, *Vienna Yearbook of Population Research 2008*, 89–102.

Asher, M. G. & Newman, D. (2001) Hong Kong and Singapore: Two approaches to the provision of pensions in Asia, *Journal of Pensions Management, 7*(2): 155–166.

Asian Development Bank (2010) *Key indicators of Asia and Pacific countries*. Online. Available https://sdbs.adb.org/sdbs/index.jsp (accessed May 25 2011).

Bade, R. & Parkin, M. (2007) *Foundations of macroeconomics*, (4th ed.). Boston, MA: Addison Wesley.

Bailey, C. A. (2007) *A guide to qualitative field research*, London: Pine Forge Press.

Becker, G. S. (1960) *An economic analysis of fertility, in NBER demographic and economic change in developing countries*, Princeton, NJ: Princeton University Press.

Becker, G. S. (1964) *Human capital*, New York: National Bureau of Economic Research.

Becker, G. S. & Lewis, G. (1973) On the interaction between the quantity and quality of children, *Journal of Political Economy*, 81: 279–288.

Becker, G. S. & Tomes, N. (1979) An equilibrium theory of the distribution of income and intergenerational mobility, *Journal of Political Economy*, 87: 1153–1189.

Bercuson, K. B. (Ed.). (1995) *Singapore: a case study in rapid development*, Washington, DC: International Monetary Fund.

Berg, B. L. (2009) *Qualitative research methods for the social sciences*, Boston, MA: Pearson.

Bezanson, K. (2006) *Gender, the state, and social reproduction: household insecurity in neo-liberal times*. Toronto: University of Toronto Press.

Bittles, A. H. & Chew, Y. Y. ([1998], 2009) Eugenics and population policies. In S. S. Strickland & P. S. Shetty (Eds.), *Human biology and social inequality*, Cambridge: Cambridge University Press.

Bjorklund, A. (2006) Does family policy affect fertility? Lessons from Sweden, *Journal of Population Economics*, 19: 3–24.

Black, S. E., Devereux, P. J., & Salvanes, K. G. (2005) The more the merrier? The effect of family size and birth order on children's education, *Quarterly Journal of Economics*, 120: 669–700.

Blackford, H. (2004) Playground panopticism: ring-around-the-children, a pocketful of women, *Childhood*, 11: 227–249.

Blair-Loy, M. & Wharton, A.S. (2004) Organizational commitment and constraints on work-family policy use: Corporate Flexibility policies in a global firm. *Sociological PerspectivesI,* 47: 243–267.

Blake, J. (1981) Family Size and the quality of children, *Demography*, 18: 421–442.

—— (1989) *Family size and achievement*, Los Angeles, CA: University of California Press.

Blomqvist, H. C. (2005) *Swimming with sharks: global and regional dimensions of the Singapore economy*, Singapore: Marshall Cavendish Academic.

Bloom, D. E. & Williamson, J. G. (1998) Demographic transitions and economic miracles in emerging Asia, *The World Bank Economic Review*, *12*(3): 419–55.

Boling, P. (2008) Demography, culture and policy: Understanding Japan's low fertility, *Population and Development Review*, 43: 307–326.

Bonoli, G. (2008) The impact of social policy on fertility: Evidence from Switzerland, *Journal of European Social Policy*, 18: 64–77.

Broberg, G. & Roll-Hansen, N. (1996, 2005) *Eugenics and the welfare state, sterilization policy in Denmark, Sweden, Norway and Finland*, East Lansing: Michigan State University Press.

Brodie, J. (1997) Meso-discourses, state forms and the gendering of liberal-democratic citizenship, *Citizenship Studies*, *1*(2): 223–242.

—— (2007) Reforming social justice in neoliberal times, *Studies in Social Justice*, 1: 93–107.

Brown, M. K., Carnoy, M., Currie, E., Duster, T., Oppenheimer, D. B., Schultz, M., & Wellman, D. (2003) *Whitewashing race: The myth of a color-blind society*, Berkeley, Los Angeles: University of California Press.

Brush, L. (2002) Changing the subject: Gender and welfare regime studies, *Social Politics: International Studies in Gender, State and Society*, 9: 161–186.

Bussemaker, J. & Voet, R. (1998) Citizenship and gender: Theoretical approaches and historical legacies, *Critical Social Policy*, 18: 277–307.

Caldwell, J. C. & Caldwell B. K. (1996) Asia's demographic transition, *Asian Development Review*, *15*(1): 52–87.

Caldwell, J. C. & Schindlmayr, T. (2003) Explanations of the fertility crisis in modern societies: A search for commonalities, *Population Studies*, 57: 241–390.

Caputo, V. (2007) She's from a "good family": Performing childhood and motherhood in a Canadian private school setting, *Childhood*, 14: 173–192.

Castles, F. G. (2003) 'The world turned upside down: below replacement fertility, changing preferences and family-friendly policy in 21 OECD countries', *Journal of European Social Policy*, 13: 209–227.

Central Provident Fund (2005a) *Chairman's foreword.* Online. Available www.cpf.gov.sg/cpf_info/CPF50Ann/chairman_Mr_Koh_text.pdf (accessed July 2008).

—— (2005b) *Saving for our retirement: 50 years of CPF*, Singapore: SNP International.

—— (2008) CPF education scheme. Online. mycpf.cpf.gov.sg/CPF/News/Highlights/ednhigh.htm (accessed March 2008).

—— (2011) CPF statistics. Online. Available http://mycpf.cpf.gov.sg/CPF/About-Us/CPF-Stats/CPF_Stats2010q3.htm (accessed May 23 2011).

Chan, A. (2005) Aging in Southeast and East Asia: issues and policy directions, *Journal of Cross Cultural Gerontology*, 20: 269–284.

Chandler, A. D. Jr. (1990) *Scale and scope: The dynamics of industrial capitalism*, Cambridge, London: The Belknap Press of Harvard University Press.

Chang, K. S. (1999) Compressed modernity and its discontent: South Korean society in transition, *Economy and Society*, *28*(1): 30–55.

—— (2010a) The second modern condition? Compressed modernity as internalized reflexive cosmopolitization, *The British Journal of Sociology* 61: 444–464.

—— (2010b) Individualization without individualism: Compressed modernity and obfuscated family crisis in East Asia, *Journal of Intimate and Public Spheres* 1: 23–29.

Chang, K. S. & Song, M.-Y. (2010) The stranded individualizer under compressed modernity: South Korean women in individualization without individualism, *British Journal of Sociology*, *61*(3): 539–564.

Cheung, P. (1989) Beyond demographic transition: industrialisation and population change in Singapore, *Asia-Pacific Population Journal*, 4: 35–48.

Chew, M. (1994) Human rights in Singapore: perceptions and problems, *Asian Survey*, 34: 933–948.

Chin, T. (2000) Sixth grade madness: parental emotion work in private high school application process, *Journal of Contemporary Ethnography*, 29: 124–163.

Choe, M. K. (2006) Modernization, gender roles and marriage behaviour in South Korea. In Y.-S. Chang and S. H. Lee (Eds.), *Transformations in twentieth century Korea*, London: Routledge.

Chua, B. H. (1995) *Communitarian ideology and democracy in Singapore*, London: Routledge.

—— (1999, May) *Global economy/immature policy: Current crisis in Southeast Asia*. Paper presented at the World Academy for Local Government and Democracy Conference, Global Flows/Local Fissures: Urban Antagonisms Revisited, Istanbul, Turkey.

—— (2000) Public housing residents as clients of the state, *Housing Studies*, 15: 45–60.

—— (2007) Emerging issues in developmental welfarism in Singapore. In J. Lee and K. W. Chan (Eds.), *The crisis of welfare In East Asia*, Lanham, MD: Lexington Books.

Chua, B. H. & Tan, J. E. (1999) Singapore: Where the new middle class sets the standard. In M. Pinches (Ed.), *Culture and privilege in capitalist Asia* (pp.137–158). London: Routledge.

Cigno, A. & Ermisch, J. (1989) A microeconomic analysis of the timing of births, *European Economic Review*, 33: 737–760.

Coleman, J. (1988) Social capital in the creation of human capital, *The American Journal of Sociology*, 94: S95–S120.

Connelly, M. (2008). *Fatal Misconception: The struggle to control world population*, Cambridge, MA and London: The Belknap Press of Harvard University Press.

Conover, P. J., Crewe, I. M., & Searing, D. D. (1991) The nature of citizenship in the United States and Great Britain: Empirical comments on theoretical themes, *Journal of Politics*, 53: 800–832.

Cox, H. C. (1998) The consequences of welfare reform: How conceptions of welfare rights are changing, *Journal of Social Policy*, 27: 1–16.

Cunningham, K. (2001) Father time: Flexible work arrangements and the law firm's failure of the family, *Stanford Law Review*, 53: 967–1008.

d'Addio, A. & d'Ercole, M. (2005) *Trends and determinants of fertility rates in OECD countries: The role of policies*. OECD Social, Employment and Migration (Working Paper No. 27). OECD: Paris.

Daly, M. (2010) *Welfare*, Cambridge: Polity Press.

Desforges, L., Jones, R., & Woods, M. (2005) New geographies of citizenship, *Citizenship Studies*, 9: 439–451.

DeTray, D. N. (2001) Child quality and the demand for children, *Journal of Political Economy*, 81(2): S71–S95.

Downey, D. (1995) When bigger is not better; family size, parental resources and children's educational performance, *American Sociological Review*, 60: 746–761.

Drakakis-Smith, D. & Graham, E. (1996) Shaping the nation state: Ethnicity, class and the new population policy in Singapore, *International Journal of Population Geography*, 2: 69–89.

Dwyer, P. (1998) Conditional citizens? Welfare rights and responsibilities in the late 1990s, *Critical Social Policy*, *18*(4): 519–543.

—— (2002) Making sense of social citizenship: Some user views on the welfare rights and responsibilities, *Critical Social Policy*, 22: 273–299.

Eaton, S. C. (2003) If you can use them: flexibility policies, organizational commitment and perceived performance, *Industrial Relations*, 42: 145–167.

East-West Center (2008) *Asia's aging population*. Online. Available http://www.eastwest center.org/fileadmin/stored/misc/FuturePop08Aging.pdf (accessed May 22 2011).

Economic Development Board (2007) *Singapore: Destination of choice. A look at the country's IHQ operations*, Singapore: The Government of Singapore.

Esping-Andersen, G. (1990) *The three worlds of welfare capitalism*, Princeton, NJ: Princeton University Press.

—— (2001) *A welfare state of the 21st century*, Tokyo: Sakurai Shoten.

Evans, J. M. (2002) Work/family reconciliation, gender wage equity and occupational segregation: The role of firms and public policy, *Canadian Public Policy*, 28: 187–216.

Faulks, K. (1998) *Citizenship in modern Britain*, Edinburgh: Edinburgh University Press.

—— (2000a) *Political sociology: A critical introduction*, Edinburgh: Edinburgh University Press.

—— (2000b) *Citizenship,* London: Routledge.

France, A. (1894) *Le lys rouge*, Paris: Calmann-Levy.

Galor, O. & Moav, O. (2002) Natural selection and the origin of economic growth, *Quarterly Journal of Economics*, 17: 1133–1191.

Gauthier, A. (2007) The Impact of family policies on fertility in industrialized countries: A review of the literature, *Population Research and Policy Review,* 16: 323–46.

Gauthier, A. & Hatzius, J. (1997) Family benefits and fertility: An econometric analysis, *Population Studies*, 51: 295–306.

George, G. (2010) Control-shift: The internet and political change in Singapore. In T. Chong (Ed.), *Management of success: Singapore revisited* (pp.257–271). Singapore: Institute of Southeast Asian Studies.

Georgellis, Y. & Wall, H. (1992) The fertility effect of dependent tax exemptions: estimates for the United States, *Applied Economics*, 24: 1139–1145.

Glass, J. & Riley, L. (1998) Family responsive policies and employee retention following childbirth, *Social Forces*, 76: 1401–1435.

Goodman, R., White G., & Kwon, K.J. (Eds.). (1998) *The East Asian welfare model: Welfare orientalism and the state,* London, New York: Routledge.

Gough, I., Wood, G., Barrientos, A., Bevan, P., Davis, P., & Room, G. (Eds.). (2004) *Insecurity and welfare regimes in Asia, Africa, and Latin America: Social policy in development contexts*, Cambridge: Cambridge University Press.

Graham, E. (1995) Singapore in the 1990s: Can population policies reverse the demographic transition, *Applied Geography*, 15: 219–232.

Graham, E., Teo, P., Yeoh, B., & Levy, S. (2002) Reproducing the Asian family across the generations: "Tradition", gender and expectations in Singapore, *Asia-Pacific Population Journal*, 17: 61–86.

Gu, B. (2009) The arrival of low fertility in China. In G. Jones, P. T. Straughan, & A, Chan (Eds.), *Ultra-low fertility in Pacific Asia: Trends, causes and policy issues*, London, New York: Routledge.

Gubhaju, B. B. & Moriki-Durand, Y. (2003) Below replacement fertility in East and Southeast Asia: Consequences and policy responses, *Journal of Population Research*, 20: 1–18.

Guo, G. & VanWey, L. K. (1999) Sibship size and intellectual development: Is the relationship casual? *American Sociological Review*, *64*(2): 169–187.

Haas, L. & Hwang, P. (1995) Company culture and men's usage of family leave benefits in Sweden, *Family Relations*, 44: 28–36.

Hakim, C. (2003) A new approach to explaining fertility patterns: Preference theory, *Population and Development Review*, 29: 349–374.

Hall, T. & Williamson, H. (1999) *Citizenship and community*, Leicester: Youth Work Press.

Hamilton, B. E., Martin, J. A., & Ventura, S. J. (2007) Births: Preliminary data for 2006. Online. Available http://www.cdc.gov/nchs/data/nvsr/nvsr56/nvsr56_07.pdf (accessed May 22 2011).

Handler, J. F. (2003) Social citizenship and workfare in the US and Western Europe: from status to contract, *Journal of European Social Policy*, 13: 229–243.

Haney, L. (1996) Homeboys, babies, men in suits: The state and the reproduction of male domination, *American Sociological Review*, 61: 759–778.

Hays, S. (1996) *The cultural contradictions of motherhood*, New Haven, CT: Yale University Press.

Hill, M. & Lian, K. F. (1995) *The politics of nation building and citizenship in Singapore*, London: Routledge.

Ho, K. L. (2010) Political consolidation in Singapore: Connecting the party, the government and the expanding state. In T. Chong (Ed.), *Management of success: Singapore revisited*. Singapore: Institute of Southeast Asian Studies.

Hochschild, A. (2003) *The commercialization of intimate life: Notes from home and work*, San Francisco, Los Angeles: University of California Press.

Holliday, I. (2000) Productivist welfare capitalism: Social policy in East Asia, *Political Studies*, 48: 706–723.

—— (2003) Health care. In I. Holliday and P. Wilding (Eds.), *Welfare capitalism in East Asia: Social policy in the tiger economies* (pp. 70–98). Basingstoke: Palgrave Macmillan.

—— (2005) East Asian social policy in the wake of the financial crisis: Farewell to productivism?, *Policy and Politics*, 33: 145–162.

Holliday, I. & Wilding, P. (Eds.). (2004) *Welfare capitalism in East Asia: Social policy in the tiger economies*, Palgrave: London.

Hu, Y.W. (2008, August 26) High inflation for the first half of the year: lower-income families were hit harder, *Lianhe Zaobao*, pp. A1.

Inland Revenue Authority of Singapore (2008) Income Tax Rates. Available http://www.iras.gov.sg/irasHome/page04.aspx?id=1190 (accessed June 2008)

International Herald Tribune (2009, September 30) Singapore wealth fund says investments fell 20% in year. Online. http://www.nytimes.com/2009/09/30/business/global/30fund.html

International Labour Organization (2006) Facts on Labor Migration. Available http://www.ilo.org/public/libdoc/ilo/2006/106B09_492_engl.pdf (accessed May 29 2011).

International Monetary Fund (2011) World Economic Outlook Database. Online. Available http://www.imf.org/external/pubs/ft/weo/2011/01/weodata/weorept.aspx?pr.x=6&pr.y=1&sy=2008&ey=2010&scsm=1&ssd=1&sort=country&ds=.&br=1&c=158%2C576%2C111&s=NGDPDPC&grp=0&a= (accessed September 24 2011)

Isin, E.F. (Ed.). (2008) *Recasting the social in citizenship*. Toronto: University of Toronto Press.

Isin, E., Brodie, J., Juteau, D., & Stasiulis, D. (2008) Recasting the social in citizenship. In I. Engin (Ed.), *Recasting the social in citizenship* (pp. 3–19). Toronto: University of Toronto Press.

Isin, E. F., Nyers, P., & Turner, B. S. (2008) *Citizenship between past and future*, London: Routledge.

Jacobs, D. (2000) Low public expenditures on social welfare: Do East Asian countries have a secret? *International Journal of Social Welfare*, *9*(1): 2–16.

Joesch, J. (1997) Paid leave and the timing of women's employment before and after birth, *Journal of Marriage and Family*, 59: 1008–1021.

Jones, G. (2004) The demography of disadvantage, *Journal of Population Research*, 21: 107–126.

Jones, G., Straughan P.T., & Chan A. (2009) Very low fertility in Pacific Asian countries. In G. Jones, P.T. Straughan, & A. Chan (Eds.), *Ultra-low fertility in Pacific Asia: Trends, causes and policy issues* (pp. 1–22). London, New York: Routledge.

—— (Eds.). (2009) *Ultra-low fertility in Pacific Asia: Trends, causes and policy issues.* London, New York: Routledge.

Joppke, C. (2008) Transformation of citizenship: Status, rights, identity. In E. F. Isin, P. Nyers, & B. S. Turner (Eds.), *Citizenship between past and future*, New York: Routledge.

Kang, T. (2005) *Creating educational dreams: The Intersection of ethnicity, families and schools*, Singapore: Marshall Cavendish Academic.

Kee, W. F. & Loh, M. (1974) Singapore, *Studies in Family Planning*, 5: 163–165.

Kee, W. F. & Saw, S. H. (1975) Knowledge, attitudes and practice of family planning in Singapore, *Studies in Family Planning*, 6: 109–112.

Kim, S. (2000) *East Asia and globalization*, New York: Rowman & Littlefield Publishers.

Kim, Y. I. A. (2007) *Impact of birth subsidies on fertility: Empirical study of allowance for newborn children, a pronatal policy*. Online. Available http://home.uchicago.edu/~kimyia/Kim%20(2007).pdf (accessed September 2009).

Kirk, D. (1980) Forward. In S.-H. Saw *Population control for zero growth in Singapore*. Oxford, New York, Melbourne: Oxford University Press.

Kohlwe, H.P., Billari, F.C., & Ortega J.A. (2002) The emergence of lowest-low fertility in Europe during the 1990s, *Population and Development Review, 28*(4): 641–680.

Krugman, P. (2009, November 1) Too little of a good thing, Op-ed, *The New York Times*.

Kwok, K. W. & Mariam, M. A. (1998) Cultivating citizenship and national identity. In L. T. Yuan and A. Mahizhnan (Eds.), *Re-engineering success*, Singapore: Oxford University Press.

Kymlicka, W. and Norman, W. (1994) Return of the citizen: A survey of recent work on citizenship theory, *Ethics*, 104: 352–381.

Lai, A. E. (2002) *Report on IPS research forum on ethnic relations in Singapore*, Singapore: The Institute of Policy Studies.

Lareau, A. (2002) Invisible Inequality: social class and childrearing in black families and white families, *American Sociological Review*, 67: 747–776.

—— (2003) *Unequal childhoods: Class, race and family life*, Berkeley, Los Angeles, London: University of California Press.

Laroque, G. & Salanie, B. (2003) *Fertility and financial incentives in France*. Online. http://www.cepr.org/meets/wkcn/3/3520/papers/laroque.pdf (accessed September 2009).

Lee, J. (2007) Deciphering productivism and developmentalism in East Asian social welfare. In J. Lee and K. W. Chan (Eds.), *The crisis of welfare in East Asia*, Lanham, MA: Lexington Books.

Lee, K. Y. (2000) *From Third World to first: The Singapore story 1965–2000*, New York: HarperCollins.

Lesthaeghe, R. (1995) The second demographic transition in Western countries: An interpretation. In K. O.Mason & A.-M. Jensen (Eds.), *Gender and family change in industrialized countries*, Oxford: Clarendon Press.

Letablier, M. T. (2003) *Fertility and family policies in France*. Online. Available http://www.ier.hit-u.ac.jp/pie/Japanese/discussionpaper/dp2003/dp160/text.pdf (accessed July 2009).

Lim, L. (February 19 2011) Lower-paid gain most from bumper payouts;

'Grow and Share' package is one of Govt's biggest bags of goodies, *The Straits Times*.

Lin, K. & Rantalaiho, M. (2003) Family policy and social order – comparing the dynamics of family policy-making in Scandinavia and Confucian Asia, *International Journal of Social Welfare*, 12: 2–13.

Lister, R. (1997/2003) *Citizenship: Feminist perspectives*, Basingstoke: Palgrave Macmillan.

—— (2007) Investing in the citizen-workers of the future: Transformations in citizenship and the state under new labour. In C. Pierson & F. G. Castles (Eds.), *The welfare state reader* (pp. 455–67). Cambridge: Polity Press.

—— (2008) Inclusive citizenship: Realizing the potential. In E. F. Isin, P. Nyers, & B. S. Turner (Eds.), *Citizenship between past and future*, London: Routledge.

Liu, H. (2003) *The transformation of Chinese society in postwar Singapore: Localizing process, regional networking, and global perspective*, Xiamen, People's Republic of China: Xiamen University Press.

—— (2011) *Brothers of a different kind? The politics of differentiating and integrating Chinese new immigrants in Singapore*. Paper presented at the International Workshop "From National to Ethnic Identifications" (University of Malaya, March 23–24 2011).

Loke, V. & Kramer R. (2009) *Singapore's Central Provident Fund: A national policy of life-long asset accounts*, Washington DC: New America Foundation. Online. Available http://www.newamerica.net/publications/policy/singapores_central_provident_fund (accessed September 22 2011).

Low, L. (2004) How Singapore's Central Provident Fund fares in social security and social policy, *Social Policy and Society*, 3: 301–10.

—— (2006) The rise of the corporate economy in Southeast Asia, *ASEAN Economic Bulletin*, 24: 282–284.

Low, L. & Aw T. C. (Eds.). (1997) *Housing a healthy, educated and wealthy nation through the CPF*, Singapore: Times Academic Press for IPS.

Low, L. & Johnston, D. M. (2003) *Singapore Inc.: Public policy options in the third millennium*, Singapore: Times Academic Press.

Lovett, L. L. (2007) *Conceiving the future: Pronatalism, reproduction, and the family in the United States 1890–1938*. Chapel Hill: The University of North Carolina Press.

Luker, K. (1997) *Dubious conceptions: the politics of teenage pregnancy*. Cambridge, MA: Havard University Press.

Marshall, T. H. (1950) *Citizenship and social class*, Chicago: University of Chicago Press.

Mau, S. (2004) Welfare regimes and the norms of social exchange, *Current Sociology*, 52: 53–74.

McCarthy, D., Mitchell, O. S., & Piggott, J. (2002) Asset rich and cash poor: retirement provision and housing policy in Singapore, *PEF*, 1: 197–222.

McDonald, P. (2000) Gender equity in theories of fertility transition, *Population and Development Review*, 26: 427–439.

—— (2002, May) *Low fertility: Unifying the theory and the demography*. Paper presented to a meeting of the Population Association of America, Atlanta, GA.

McDonald, P. & Evans A. (2002) *Family formation and risk aversion*, paper prepared for the NLC workshop 17–18 May 2002. Online. http://lifecourse.anu.edu.au/publications/Workshop1_papers/McDonald_w1.pdf (accessed May 22 2011).

Midgley, J. & Tang, K. L. (2001) Social policy, economic growth and developmental welfare, *International Journal of Social Welfare*, 10: 244–252.

Milligan, K. (2002) *Quebec's baby bonus: Can public policy raise fertility*, Backgrounder, CD: Howe Institute.

Minorities at Risk Project (2004) *Chronology for Malays in Singapore*. Online. Available http://www.unhcr.org/refworld/docid/469f38d91e.html (accessed July 2008).

Ministry of Community Development, Youth and Sports (2008) Singapore's fourth periodic report to the UN Committee for the Convention on the Elimination of All Forms of Discrimination against Women. Online. Available http://www.mcys.gov.sg/MCDSFiles/Download/Fourth_Periodic_Report.pdf (accessed September 22 2011).

Ministry of Education, Singapore (2007) *Curriculum planning and development division, 2007, upper secondary social studies textbook*, Singapore: Ministry of Education.

—— (2009) Primary and Secondary Education. Online. Available http://www.moe.gov.sg/education/primary/, http://www.moe.gov.sg/education/secondary/ (accessed June 2007).

—— *Education Statistics Digest 2010*, The Government of Singapore. Online. Available http://www.moe.gov.sg/education/education-statistics-digest/ (accessed September 22 2011).

Ministry of Finance, Singapore (2002) *Strong stable families*. Online. Available http://www.mof.gov.sg/budget_2002/expendhighlights/budget_mcds.html (accessed June 2007).

—— (2003) *Strong stable families*. Online. Available http://www.mof.gov.sg/budget_2003/exp_overview/budget_mcds.html (accessed June 2007)

—— (2004) *Strong stable families*. Online. Available http://www.mof.gov.sg/budget_2004/exp_overview/exp_over_section1.5.html (accessed June 2007)

Ministry of Health, Ministerial Committee on Health Policies (1993) *Affordable health care: A white paper*, Singapore: Singapore National Printers [for] Ministry of Health.

Ministry of Manpower (2008) *Employment of Singapore citizens, permanent residents and foreigners*, Singapore: The Government of Singapore.

—— (2009) *Report on labour force in Singapore 2008*, Singapore: The Government of Singapore.

—— (2010) *Labour Force Survey* 2010. Online. Available http://www.mom.gov.sg/statistics-publications/national-labour-market-information/publications/Pages/default.aspx (accessed September 22 2011).

—— (2011a) Passes and visas. Online. Available http://www.mom.gov.sg/foreign-manpower/passes-visas/Pages/default.aspx (accessed May 12 2011).

—— (2011b) Unemployment. Online. Available http://www.mom.gov.sg/statistics-publications/national-labour-market-information/statistics/Pages/unemployment.aspx (accessed May 5 2011).

Moav, O. (2005) Cheap children and the persistence of poverty, *Economic Journal*, 115: 88–110.

Monetary Authority of Singapore (2009) *Singapore's growing income disparities: Causes, consequences, and policy options*. Online. Available http://www.mas.gov.sg/resource/

eco_research/eco_education/Esss2007/Pre_Uni_2nd_Ee%20Kuan.pdf (accessed September 25 2011).

—— (2011). Official foreign reserves. Online. Available http://www.mas.gov.sg/data_room/reserves_statistics/Official_Foreign_Reserves.html (accessed April 26 2011).

Morgan, D. L. (1997) *Focus Groups as qualitative research*, Thousand Oaks, CA: Sage Publications.

Mydan, S. (May 8 2011) Opposition makes inroads in Singapore, *New York Times.*

Myrskyla, M., Kohler, H.-P., & Billari, F. C. (2009) Advances in development reverse fertility declines, *Nature*, *460*(6): 741–743.

National Population and Talent Division (2009) Population in brief 2009. Online. Available https://www.nptd.gov.sg/content/NPTD/news/_jcr_content/par_content/download_0/file.res/Population%20in%20Brief%202009.pdf (accessed May 22 2011).

—— (2011a) Comparison of marriage and parenthood packages: 2001, 2004, and 2008. Online. Available https://www.nptd.gov.sg/content/NPTD/news/_jcr_content/par_content/download_20/file.res/Comparison%20of%20Marriage%20and%20Parenthood%20Packages%20-%202001%202004%20and%202008.pdf (accessed May 22 2011).

—— (2011b) Organisation chart. Online. Available https://www.nptd.gov.sg/content/NPTD/about_nps.html#chart (accessed May 27 2011)

Ness, G. D. & Ando, H. (1984) *The land is shrinking: Population planning in Asia,* Baltimore, London: The Johns Hopkins University Press.

Ness, G. D. & Low, M. M. (2000) *Five cities: Modelling Asian urban population-environment dynamics*, Oxford: Oxford University Press.

Newman, D. M. (2004) *Exploring the architecture of everyday life*, Newbury Park, CA: Pine Forge Press.

Neyer, G. (2003) Family policies and low fertility in Western Europe, *Journal of Population and Social Security (Population)*, Supplement to Volume 1: 46–93.

Ochiai, E. (2010) Reconstruction of Intimate and public spheres in Asian modernity: familialism and beyond', *Journal of Intimate and Public Spheres*, 1: 2–22.

Offe, C. (1984) *Contradictions of the welfare state*, London: Hutchinson.

Ogawa, N., Retherford, R. D., & Matsukura, R. (2006) Demographics of the Japanese family: entering unchartered territory. In M. Rebick and A. Takenaka (Eds.), *The changing Japanese family*, London: Routledge.

Oi, M. (2010) Singapore's tough balancing act on immigration. *Asia Business Report*. BBC World. Online. Available http://www.bbc.co.uk/news/business-11100813 (accessed March 17 2011).

Olah, L. (2003) Gendering fertility: second births in Sweden and Hungary, *Population and Policy Review*, 22: 171–200.

Orloff, A. S. (1993) Gender and the social rights of citizenship: The comparative analysis of gender relations and welfare states, *American Sociological Review*, 58: 303–328.

Osman-Gani, A. M. (2004) Human capital development in Singapore: An analysis of national policy perspectives, *Advances in Developing Human Resources*, 6: 276–287.

Palen, J. J. (1986) Fertility and eugenics: Singapore's population policies, *Population Research and Policy Review*, 5: 3–14.

Pateman, C. (1988) *The sexual contract*, Cambridge: Polity.

Pereira, A. A. (2008) Manufacturing human resources: The role of social investment state. In K. F. Lian & C. K. Tong (Eds.), *Social policy in post-industrial Singapore*, Leiden: Brill.

Plant, R. (1991) Social rights and the reconstruction of welfare. In G. Andrews (Ed.), *Citizenship*, London: Lawrence & Wishart.

Population Division, Department of Economic and Social Affairs, United Nations. (2004) *World fertility report* 2003, New York: United Nations.

Population Reference Bureau (2010) Total Fertility Rate (TFR), Online. Available http://www.prb.org/Datafinder/Topic/Bar.aspx?sort=v&order=a&variable=93 (accessed May 22 2011).

Quah, S. R. (1998) *Family in Singapore: Sociological perspectives*, Singapore: Times Academic Press.

—— (2009) *Families in Asia: Home and kin*. London: Routledge.

Ramesh, M. (2000) *Welfare capitalism in Southeast Asia*, Basingstoke: Palgrave.

—— (2004) *Social policy in the East and Southeast Asia: Education, health, housing and income maintenance*, London: RoutledgeCurzon.

Retherford, R. D. & Sewell, W. H. (1991) Birth order and intelligence: Further tests of the confluence model, *American Sociological Review*, 56: 141–158.

Risse, L. (2006, December) Determinants of maternity leave provisions in Australia and the effects on fertility: An application of the Heckprobit Selection Model. In K. Reed (Convener) *ASCPRI Social science methodology conference*, Sydney, Australia.

Ritchie, J. & Spencer L. (2002) Qualitative data analysis for applied policy research. In A. M. Huberman and M. B. Miles (Eds.), *The Qualitative Researcher's Companion*, Thousand Oaks, CA: Sage Publications.

Rodan, G. (1989) *The political economy of Singapore's industrialization: National state and international capital*, Basingstoke: Macmillan.

—— (2004) The coming challenge to Singapore Inc, *Far Eastern Economic Review*, December, 168 (1): 51–54. Online. Available http://www.singapore-window.org/sw04/041200fe.htm (accessed September 24 2011).

Rodan, G., K. Hewison, & R. Robison (Eds.). (2006) *The political economy of South-East Asia: Markets, power and contestation*, Oxford: Oxford University Press.

Ronsen, M. (2004) Fertility and public policies: Evidence from Norway and Finland, *Demographic Research*, 10: 146–170.

Rostgaard, T. (2004) Family support policy in Central and Eastern Europe: A decade and a half of transition. *Early childhood and family policy series No.8.* Online. Available http://unesdoc.unesco.org/images/0013/001337/133733e.pdf (accessed July 2009).

Sandhu, K. S. & Wheatley, P. (1989) *Management of success: The moulding of modern Singapore*, Singapore: Institute of Southeast Asian Studies.

Saw, S.-H. (1980) *Population control for zero growth in Singapore*. Oxford, New York, Melbourne: Oxford University Press.

—— (1990) *Changes in the fertility policy of Singapore*. Singapore: Times Academic Press for IPS.

—— (2005) *Population policies and programmes in Singapore*, Singapore: Institute of Southeast Asian Studies.

—— (2007) *The Population of Singapore* (2nd ed.). Pasir Panjang, Singapore: Institute of Southeast Asian Studies.

Saxonberg, S. & Szelewa D. (2007) The continuing legacy of the communist legacy? The development of family policies in Poland and the Czech Republic, *Social Politics: International Studies in Gender, State and Society*, 14: 351–379.

Schild, V. (2000) Neo-liberalism's new gendered market citizens: The "civilizing" dimension of social programmes in Chile, *Citizenship Studies*, *4*(3): 275–305.

Schuck, P. H. (2002) Liberal citizenship. In E. F. Isin & B. S. Turner (Eds.), *Handbook of citizenship studies*, Los Angeles, London, New Delhi, Singapore: Sage.

Shkolnikov, V., Andreev, E., Houle, R., & Vaupel, J. (2007) The concentration of reproduction in cohorts of women in Europe, *Population and Development Review*, 33: 67–99.

Siltanen, J. (2002) Paradise paved? Reflections on the fate of social citizenship in Canada, *Citizenship Studies*, *6*(4): 395–414.

Singapore Department of Statistics (2000) Glossary: Census 2000 concepts and definitions. Online. Available http://webcache.googleusercontent.com/search?q=cache:bwOTr7O6n9EJ:www.singstat.gov.sg/statsres/glossary/population.html+permanent+resident+definition+singapore&cd=16&hl=en&ct=clnk&gl=sg&source=www.google.com.sg (accessed May 22 2011).

—— (2001). Singapore census of population 2000. Online. Available http://www.singstat.gov.sg/pubn/census.html (accessed May 29 2011).

—— (2002, June) Income Distribution and Inequality Measures in Singapore, paper presented at *Chinese population and socioeconomic studies: Utilizing the 2000/2001 round census data*, Hong Kong University of Science and Technology in Hong Kong SAR.

—— (2003) *Key indicators of the household expenditure survey, 1988–2003*, Singapore: The Government of Singapore.

—— (2006a) *General household survey 2005*, Singapore: The Government of Singapore.

—— (2006b) *Trends in dual-career couples, 2005*, Singapore: The Government of Singapore.

—— (2008) *Population trends 2008*, Singapore: The Government of Singapore.

—— (2009a) *Population trends 2009*, Singapore: The Government of Singapore.

—— (2009b) *Key household income trends 2008*. Online. Available http://www.straitstimes.com/STI/STIMEDIA/pdf/20090120/op-s15.pdf (accessed May 25 2011).

—— (2009c) *Report on the Household Expenditure Survey 2007/2008*. Online. Available http://www.singstat.gov.sg/pubn/hhld/hes2007.pdf (accessed September 24 2011).

—— (2010a) *Population trends 2010*, Singapore: The Government of Singapore.

—— (2010b) *Foreign equity investment in Singapore, 2008*. Singapore: The Government of Singapore.

—— (2010c) Key annual indicators. Online. Available http://www.singstat.gov.sg/stats/keyind.html (accessed May 29 2011).

—— (2011a) Census of population 2010 statistical release 1: Demographic characteristics, education, language and religion. Online. Available http://www.singstat.gov.sg/pubn/popn/c2010sr1.html (accessed May 22 2011).

—— (2011b) *Press release: Household income increased in 2010*. Singapore: The Government of Singapore.

—— (2011c) Time series on annual GDP at current market prices. Online. Available http://www.singstat.gov.sg/stats/themes/economy/hist/gdp2.html (accessed May 5 2011)

—— (2011d) Time series on per capita GDP at current market prices. Available http://www.singstat.gov.sg/stats/themes/economy/hist/gdp.html (accessed May 5 2011).

—— (2011e) Key indicators on gender. Online. Available http://www.singstat.gov.sg/stats/themes/people/gender.pdf (accessed May 5 2011).

—— various years. *Yearbook of statistics*.

—— various years. *Singapore consumer price index*.

Somers, M. (2008) *Genealogies of citizenship: markets, statelessness, and the right to have rights*. Cambridge: Cambridge University Press.

Steelman, L. C. (1985) A tale of two variables: A review of the intellectual consequences of sibship size and birth order, *Review of Educational Research*, 55: 353–386.

Stein, R. (2007, December 21) U.S fertility rate hits 35 year high, stabilizing population, *The Washington Post*, p. A11.

Stewart, K. & Huerta, C. (2006) *Reinvesting in children? Policies for the very young in Southeast Europe and the CIS*. Innocenti (Working Paper, 2006–01). Florence, Italy: UNICEF Innocenti Research Center.

Straughan, P. (2008) Family policies: Interface of gender, work, and the sacredization of child. In K. F. Lian and C. K. Tong (Eds.), *Social policy in post-industrial Singapore*, Leiden: Brill.

Straughan, P. T., Chan, A., & Jones, G. (2009) From population control to fertility promotion: A case study of family policies and fertility trends in Singapore. In G. Jones, P. T. Straughan, & A. Chan (Eds.), *Ultra-low fertility in Pacific Asia: Trends, causes and policy issues*, New York: Routledge.

Suarez, S. (2009) Economic and fertility policies in an era of globalization: A comparison of Ireland and Singapore, *New Global Studies*, 3: 1–26.

Sun, H.-L. (2009) Re-producing citizens: Gender, employment, and work–family balance policies in Singapore, *Journal of Workplace Rights*, *14*(3): 351–374.

—— (2010) From citizen-duty to state-responsibility: Globalization and nationhood in Singapore, *New Global Studies*, *4*(3): 1–26.

—— Forthcoming. Social reproduction and the limits of a neo-liberal approach to citizenship, *Citizenship Studies*, 16 (2).

Sung, J. (2006) *Explaining the economic success of Singapore*, Cheltenham: Edward Elgar.

Sussman, S., Burton, D., Dent, C.W., & Stacy, A.W. (1991) Use of focus groups in developing an adolescent tobacco use cessation program: Collective norm effects, *Journal of Applied Social Psychology*, 23: 1772–1882.

Tan, L. & Goh, C.B. (2008) The development of university education in Singapore. In L.S. Kong (Ed.), *Toward a better future: Education and training for economic development in Singapore since 1965*, Washington, DC: The World Bank; Singapore: National Institute of Education.

Tan, L. (2010) The dollars and sense of parenthood: bringing a child up to tertiary education level can cost new parents between $190k and $700k. *The Straits Times*, July 4 2010.

Tan, T. H. & Asmani A. (March 13 2004) Baby debate: Words that don't bear repeating, *The Straits Times*.

Taylor-Gooby, P. (1991) Welfare state regimes and welfare citizenship, *Journal of European Social Policy*, 1: 93–105.

Teo, P. & Yeoh, B. (1999) Interweaving the public and the private: women's responses to population policy shifts in Singapore, *International Journal of Population Geography*, 5: 79–96.

Teo, Y. Y. (2010) Shaping the Singapore family, producing the state and society, *Economy and Society*, *39*(3): 337–359.

Tham, S. C. (1989) The perception and practice of education. In K. S. Sandhu and P. Wheatley (Eds.), *Management of success: The Moulding of Singapore,* Singapore: Institute of Southeast Asian Studies.

Thang, L. L. (2005) Private matters, public concern: procreation issues in Singapore, *The Japanese Journal of Population*, 3: 76–108.

The Democratic Party of Japan (2009) *2009 Change of government, the Democratic Party of Japan's platform for government: Putting people's lives first*. Online. Available http://www.dpj.or.jp/english/manifesto/manifesto2009.pdf (accessed September 22 2011).

The Institute of Policy Studies (2011, March 16) T*he Bukit Timah dialogues: Singapore's population challenge*. Online. Available http://www.spp.nus.edu.sg/docs/Singapore%20 Experience/BTD/20110316_BTD_Tay_Choon_Hong.pdf (accessed May 22 2011).

Thorne, B. (1999) Pick up time at Oakdale Elementary School: Work and family from the vantage points of children. Working and occasional papers, Berkeley Center for Working Families.

Tremewan, C. (1994) *The Political economy of social control in Singapore*, New York: St. Martin's Press.

—— (1998) Welfare and governance: Public housing under Singapore's party-state. In R. Goodman, G. White, & H.-J. Kwon (Eds.), *The East Asian welfare model: Welfare orientalism and the state.* London, New York: Routledge.

Turnbull, C. M. (2009) *A history of modern Singapore, 1819–2005*, Singapore: National University of Singapore Press.

Turner, B. S. (2001) The erosion of citizenship, *British Journal of Sociology*, 52: 189–209.

—— (2010) Ralf Dahrendorf on citizenship and life chances, *Citizenship Studies*, *14*(2): 237–244.

Tversky, A. & Kahneman, D. (1981) The framing of decisions and the psychology of choice, *Science*, *211*(4481): 453–58.

United Nations (2002) *World population aging: 1950–2050.* Online. Available http://www.un.org/esa/population/publications/worldageing19502050/ (accessed May 22 2011).

—— (2010) World population to reach 10 billion by 2100 if fertility in all countries converges to replacement level. Online. Available http://esa.un.org/unpd/wpp/other-information/Press_Release_WPP2010.pdf (accessed September 24 2011).

—— (2011a) *World population prospects: The 2010 revision.* Online. Available http://esa.un.org/wpp/Other-Information/faq.htm (accessed May 22 2011).

—— (2011b) *World population to reach 10 billion by 2100 if fertility in all countries converges to replacement level.* Online. Available http://esa.un.org/unpd/wpp/other-information/Press_Release_WPP2010.pdf (accessed May 22 2011).

Van de Kaa, D.J. (1987) Europe's second demographic transition, *Population Bulletin 42*(1), Washington: Population Reference Bureau.

Verweij, M. & Pelizzo, R. (2009) Singapore: Does authoritarianism pay? *Journal of Democracy*, 20: 18–32.

Vikat, A. (2004) Women's labour force attachment and childbearing in Finland, *Demographic Research Special Collection*, 3: 175–211.

Wan, D. & Tak K. H. (2008) The changing face of human resource management in Singapore. In C. Rowley and S. Abdul-Rahman (Eds.), *The changing face of management in South East Asia*, New York: Routledge.

Wan, F. K. & Loh, M. (1979) Fertility policies and the National Family Planning and Population Programme. In P. S. J. Chen & J. T. Fawcett (Eds.), *Public policy and population change in Singapore*, New York: Population Council.

Wee, V. (1995) Children, population policy, and the state in Singapore. In S. Stevens (Ed.), *Children and the politics of culture*, Princeton: Princeton University Press.

Wharton, A. S., Chivers, S. & Blair-Loy M. (2008) Use of formal and informal work–family policies on the digital assembly line, *Work and Occupations*, 35: 327–350.

White, G. & Goodman, R. (1998) Welfare orientalism and the search for an East Asian welfare model, in R. Goodman, G. White, & H. J. Kwon (Eds.), *The East Asian welfare model: Welfare orientalism and the state*, New York: Routledge.

Whittington, L., Alm, J., & Peter, H. (1990) Fertility and the personal exemption: implicit pronatalist policy in the United States, *The American Economic Review*, 80: 545–556.

Wong, C.-K., Wang, K. Y.-T., & Kaun, P.-Y. (2009) Social citizenship rights and the welfare circle dilemma: Attitudinal findings of two Chinese societies, *Asian Social Work and Policy Review*, *3*(1): 51–62.

Wong, C.-K. & Wong, K. Y. (2005) Expectations and practice in social citizenship: some insights from an attitude survey in a Chinese society, *Social Policy and Administration*, *39*(1): 19–34.

Wong, T. & Yeoh, B. (2003) Fertility and the family: An overview of pro-natalist population policies in Singapore. (Research Paper Series No. 12). Asian MetaCentre, National University of Singapore, Singapore.

World Bank (2011) Fertility rate, total. Online. Available http://data.worldbank.org/indicator/SP.DYN.TFRT.IN (accessed May 25 2011).

Yamaguchi, K. & Lee, W. (2008) On the relationship between female labor-force participation and total fertility rate among OECD countries: Two roles of work–family balance. In American Sociological Association Annual Meeting, Boston.

Yap, M. T. (2009) Ultra-low fertility in Singapore. In G. Jones, P. T. Straughan, & A. Chan (Eds.), *Ultra-low fertility in Pacific Asia: Trends, causes and policy issues*, New York: Routledge.

Yardley, J. (2008, February 28) China wants gradual shift away from its one-child policy, *International Herald Tribune*, p.3.

Young, I. M. (1989) Polity and group difference: a critique of the ideal of universal citizenship, *Ethics* 99 (2): 250–274.

Zajonc, R. B. & Markus, G. B. (1975) Birth order and intellectual development, *Psychological Review*, 82: 74–88.

Index

In this index **bold type** indicates figures and tables; appendices are indicated by a.; notes by n.